Praise f

"*The Yogi's Way* is a deeply Reema Datta's rich family tradition and decades of experience on and off the mat. With humility and gentleness, Reema authentically invites you to transform from within, guiding you to build a profound community of sacred friends as you evolve step-by-step on your spiritual path."

— **Ananta Ripa Ajmera**, award-winning and bestselling author of *The Ayurveda Way* and *The Way of the Goddess*

"In this luminous guide, Reema Datta leads us through a program of awakening that is both gentle and empowering. Her teachings draw on thousands of years of yogic wisdom and are translated to fit the shape of current Western conditions and lift us from the pervasive spell of anxiety, depression, and fear of not being enough. Highly recommended."

— **Mirabai Starr**, author of *Wild Mercy* and *Ordinary Mysticism*

"*The Yogi's Way* reveals the magical and transformative power of Reema Datta's teachings. Her wisdom has transformed my life for the better, and I am sure it will do just that for you too. A poetic, profound, and beautiful read."

— **Zainab Salbi**, author and founder of Women for Women International and Daughters for Earth

"With wisdom both ancient and modern, Reema Datta offers a practical and poetic pathway to finding your *svadharma* — your unique gifts and purpose. *The Yogi's Way* is a true treasure, rich in philosophy, mantra, ritual, and powerful practices to help you skillfully navigate these challenging times. I will refer to it often as a yogini, a yoga teacher, and a student of life. Bravo!"

— **Leza Lowitz**, author of *Yoga Heart: Lines on the Six Perfections*

"Reema Datta speaks from the heart and teaches from experience. Her dedication and belief in the transformative power of yoga are powerful and infectious. Spend a few moments with her words. It will feel like you are being warmly received into the magical world of yoga."

— **Simon Park**, founder of Liquid Flow Yoga

"Living in the USA and India and teaching worldwide, Reema Datta has dedicated her whole life to understanding how yoga, on its ever-expanding trail as 'soul work,' can bring people well-being, peace, joy, true freedom, and fulfillment of personal destiny. As a tool for personal authority and personal responsibility leading to universal responsibility, *The Yogi's Way* is her unique and innovative expression and interpretation of this ancestral knowledge. Reema's book and teachings beautifully add to the current positive, revolutionary effect of yoga on our entire world."

— **Danny Paradise** (DannyParadise.com), international yoga and martial arts teacher, musician, composer, filmmaker, performance artist, and human rights activist

"As a male teacher and practitioner, I am deeply touched by Reema Datta's book, which bridges East and West and offers her profound, sensitive, and activistic female approach to yoga. This book will be a gift to the yoga community."

— **Athanasios Koutsogiannis**, founder of Zorba Yoga

"Reema Datta bridges the gap between her traditional yoga upbringing and the practical usage of yoga in the modern context. I couldn't recommend this book more."

— **Adam Keen**, yoga teacher and founder of Keen on Yoga platform and podcast

"Those who experience yoga with Reema will be touched by her presence and offerings, as have I."

— **Sting**

"Reema is that rare person who radiates purity of essence and intention and has the ability to inspire these qualities in others just by entering the room. I know because I've experienced it."

— **Edie Brickell**

THE YOGI'S WAY

THE YOGI'S WAY®

Transform Your Mind, Health, and Reality

REEMA DATTA

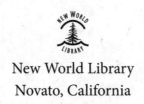

New World Library
Novato, California

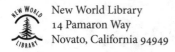 New World Library
14 Pamaron Way
Novato, California 94949

The material in this book is intended for education. It is not meant to take the place of diagnosis and treatment by a qualified medical practitioner or therapist. No expressed or implied guarantee of the effects of the use of the recommendations can be given nor liability taken. Some names and identifying characteristics have been changed to protect privacy.

The Yogi's Way® and Heal Yourself Now® are registered trademarks of Reema Datta's Yatri, LLC.

Text design by Tona Pearce Myers

Library of Congress Cataloging-in-Publication data is available.

First printing, February 2025
ISBN 978-1-60868-940-8
Ebook ISBN 978-1-60868-941-5
Printed in Canada

10   9   8   7   6   5   4   3   2   1

New World Library is committed to protecting our natural environment. This book is made of material from well-managed FSC®-certified forests and other controlled sources.

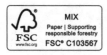

To my grandparents,
Ba, Baba, Granny, and Bapuji;
my parents,
Lata and Vasant;
and my daughter, Mila.

The mind is a wondrous power.
Our destiny in life is determined by what we do with that power.

Sri Ramana Maharshi

Each chapter in this book offers a set of practices, including mantra, meditation, visualization, breathing, or movement. To access recordings of these teachings by Reema Datta, visit:

TheYogisWay.com/thebook

CONTENTS

INTRODUCTION

A Return to Wisdom

Throughout the world, yoga is often equated with a physical practice. By contrast, its original teachings focus on the mind and consciousness. Ancient yogic wisdom offers beautiful and practical guidance on how to face and move through difficult thoughts and emotions and connect with consciousness — the deepest and most powerful part of ourselves.

Welcome to *The Yogi's Way*, where our practice centers on cultivating a direct and intimate connection with consciousness, a dimension of love and boundless possibility within us. From this space, we learn to meet the full spectrum of emotions with tenderness, curiosity, and courage. This helps us overcome the human tendency to either brush aside or be drained by uncomfortable and intense emotions such as anger, shame, or fear when they arise.

The Yogi's Way is a holistic method of yoga that integrates movement and breathing practices with yoga's original teachings on the mind and consciousness. It focuses on emotional well-being as a gateway to realizing your full potential. As mind and body open and we give our emotions the affection and care they need, their grip on us weakens, and we can rest in consciousness for longer periods. In the process, dormant creative energies stir and awaken, guiding us to discover, refine, and nurture our *svadharma* — the unique gifts we were born to contribute to the world (our purpose).

When we resist or become overly entangled with challenging emotions, they can turn into *kleshas*, the Sanskrit word for harmful thoughts and emotions. Kleshas cloud our ability to access the depths of consciousness, blocking our spiritual growth and the fulfillment of our potential. The Yoga Sutras (200 BCE) identify major kleshas as anger, attachment, delusion, pride, and fear. *The Yogi's Way* also addresses the kleshas of anxiety, depression, shame, jealousy, and loneliness, because they are so prevalent in our world today.

Our practice is not to repress our emotions or let them run our lives. Instead, we learn to face and work through our kleshas with acceptance and understanding, thereby reducing our experience of them and diminishing their harmful impacts. If kleshas go on unchecked, they can cause *granthis* — knots within the body — which lead to imbalance and potentially serious diseases.

Ancient wisdom and modern science agree on the significant impact of thoughts and emotions on physical health. Studies have shown that anger, resentment, self-pity, isolation, and distrust can create illnesses and impede recovery. Love, forgiveness, hope, and connection with community have been shown to aid health and healing. Research consistently reveals that the hormones and neurotransmitters associated with emotion can affect us physically.

Over five thousand years ago, yogis knew what scientists are discovering today: The mind has the power to destroy us or propel us to greater peace, creativity, possibility, vitality, and freedom.

As rates of anxiety, depression, low self-worth, and physical illness escalate across all demographics, *The Yogi's Way* distills essential elements of yoga philosophy and practice, offering a timely return to ancient wisdom. This journey is an invitation to develop emotional resilience, unlock creative potential, and build a life of purpose, integrity, and better overall health.

A Woman's Voice

Prominent yoga methods such as Ashtanga, Iyengar, Kundalini, Bikram, and Anusara predominantly reflect male perspectives. As I navigated my own journey of practice and learning, I longed for and sought out a woman's perspective. It's been hard to find. My female students report the same thing. It's been estimated that 72 percent of yoga practitioners in the US are women. Women consistently make up the vast majority of yoga practitioners worldwide. Yet much of the yoga we practice and teach is shaped by male perspectives.

On one hand, spirituality transcends gender. On the other, women's perspectives are indispensable. Rooted in ancestral wisdom, this book presents my interpretation of how yogic wisdom can support us in cultivating emotional well-being and living fully in our rapidly changing world. It offers guidance for practicing yoga in a holistic and healing manner.

The Yogi's Way addresses the human condition — how thoughts and emotions impact our health and reality. It reveals the profound peace and possibility we can experience when we align with our purpose and potential and live in integrity. While offering a feminine perspective, this path isn't exclusively for women. It's for anyone who has struggled with their mind and is ready to transform it from a source of bondage to one of liberation.

I was born in Maryland into a family of yogis. My parents immigrated to the US from India in 1969, seven years before my birth. From the time I was in the womb, I heard my mother sing Sanskrit mantras from the yoga tradition. They became my childhood lullabies. I learned Ayurvedic cooking and self-care rituals from my mother and grandmothers. My grandfather had a passion for yoga philosophy and wrote several books on the topic. He was my first teacher of Vedic philosophy and *pranayama* (yogic breathing techniques). My bedtime stories were renditions of classic yogic texts, such as the Bhagavad Gita and the Upanishads. My parents and grandparents translated the deep meanings behind every detail, planting seeds in my mind that the choices we make have the power to shape our world. My father's quiet and steadfast support made him the most unassuming yogi among us all.

I have been teaching yoga worldwide since 2002. I confess, in the first decade of my teaching career, I focused on the physical aspects of yoga. I love movement and taught lightly on the mind-training essentials yoga offers — until my own life abruptly shifted, and I needed those teachings myself. As one of my mentors, Manny Medina, a Native American wisdom keeper, says, "We teach best what we need to learn the most."

In 2012, my world began to fall apart. The father of my one-year-old daughter started talking about separation, expressing both his love for our daughter and his wish to live in separate households. I was devastated and heartbroken. During that time and for several years after, I intensely experienced emotions such as anger, fear, jealousy, anxiety, sorrow, shame, and isolation.

When my daughter was three years old, I made the difficult decision for the two of us to move across the country into my parents' home. There, while navigating the loss of everything that I felt defined me — my family unit, partnership, home, and career — I poured myself into the study of the original yoga texts that line my parents' bookshelves and that I had been introduced to as a child: the Vedas, Upanishads, Bhagavad Gita, and Yoga Sutras. This time, I read the wisdom with the eyes of a mother, woman, and person who had experienced a deep wounding. The teachings came alive to me in a different way. My entire approach to yoga changed. I realized what had been missing in my practice: an understanding of how to face and navigate painful thoughts and emotions — specifically, kleshas.

Bear in mind that no emotion is inherently good or bad. Our emotions are often complex and challenging, yet they are an essential part of the human experience, carrying important messages for us to receive. On this path, as we learn to meet our emotions with wisdom and compassion, we experience them in healing rather than harmful ways.

Yogic wisdom texts express tremendous empathy for our human journey. There is no need to judge ourselves for experiencing any of the kleshas. It's natural to feel the full spectrum of emotions and experiences, including our resistance to pain. As we embrace ourselves wholeheartedly and learn to move through kleshas, we create space to connect with consciousness and deepen our relationship with this most limitless and liberated part of ourselves.

Yoga, Defined

Yoga was originally transmitted and preserved in the Sanskrit language. Sanskrit words are so layered with meaning and cultural context that many of them don't have an English equivalent. The words *yoga*, *mind*, *body*, and *true Self* are perfect examples.

Yoga means "to yoke" or "to join." It unites us with our true Self. But what does this even mean?

True Self

In yoga terminology, *true Self* refers to our innermost being, which is also called "consciousness." At the very depths of our being — beyond all the ups and downs of life — there is an ever-present quietness and vastness. As we learn to yoke to this part of ourselves, extraordinary things start to happen. Dormant creative energies awaken. We experience insight and vitality. We become intuitive and innovative. We come to know our *svadharma*, a Sanskrit word that means "the right action for *you*." *Svadharma* refers to our place in the world, our unique path and gifts — our purpose. After all, it is in the giving that magic happens and life becomes meaningful and joyful.

With practice, we learn to anchor ourselves in consciousness, or the true Self. From this quiet space, we can rest, restore, heal, center, and act passionately in the world. We explore our interests, contribute our gifts, and take care of our responsibilities while remaining inwardly calm and stable no matter the outcome of our actions. Whether we experience praise or criticism, profit or loss, joy or heartbreak, we are connected to an underlying space of unshakable peace and unlimited possibility.

Imagine that level of peace and freedom. It *is* possible.

So how do we connect with our true Self? What's the biggest hindrance? Our own mind.

Mind

In yoga terminology, *mind* is defined as "the storehouse of thoughts and emotions." Written in the sixth century BCE, the Taittiriya Upanishad identifies the "lower mind" as impulsive, automatic, conditioned, and reactive. By contrast, the "higher mind" is discerning and allows us to consciously respond to life in ways that are helpful instead of harmful.

According to the Yoga Sutras, the biggest obstacle to spiritual growth — that is, union with the true Self — is being bound by kleshas, which are literally translated as "mind poisons" or "destructive emotions." When the mind is clouded with kleshas, it is hard to think clearly and make good choices. I have witnessed in myself and in my students that acknowledging our kleshas and learning to work through them has helped us shift from the lower to the higher mind. From here, we make better choices, heal destructive patterns, and create a foundation inside ourselves to experience an enduring peace of mind. This directly affects our physical vitality, emotional resilience, creative energy, and ability to honor our svadharma, our purpose and potential.

Body

In the Taittiriya Upanishad, the term *body* does not only refer to the physical body. The body consists of five layers: the physical, energetic, mental (lower mind), conscious (higher mind), and bliss bodies, which we will explore in Week Three. The fact that the very definition of *body* includes the lower and higher minds reveals the profound understanding yogis had of the mind-body connection, a theme explored throughout this book. The ancient texts illuminate that our thoughts and emotions determine the state of our physical body as well as our personal reality.

Spirit and Soul

On the level of spirit, we each have unique gifts to discover, nurture, and contribute. As mentioned above, the Sanskrit word for this is *svadharma* (स्वधर्म). Spirit yearns to express these unique attributes. On a soul level, we are identical. Each of us carries the same infinite light and potential as the Universe. The Sanskrit word for this is *Atman* (आत्मन्).

A spiritual warrior is someone who has cultivated the qualities to honor who they truly are in their spirit and their soul: a fierce determination, an indomitable will, courage, honesty, focus, discipline, daring, patience, and perseverance. In this book, we will develop these qualities.

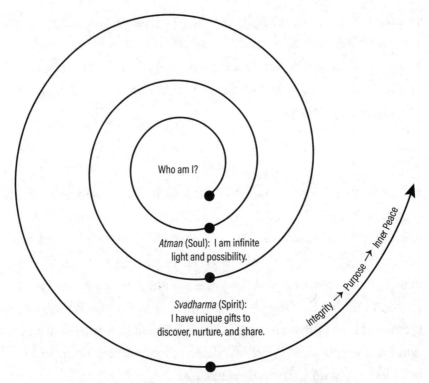

Who am I?

Atman (Soul): I am infinite
light and possibility.

Svadharma (Spirit):
I have unique gifts to
discover, nurture, and share.

Integrity → Purpose → Inner Peace

Spiritual Warrior: I cultivate courage, honesty, and discipline
to honor my soul and spirit.

FIGURE 1: The Yogi's Way to inner peace and freedom.

Sources

My family follows the tradition of Advaita Vedanta, which carries
the original teachings of yoga. These teachings, often referred to
as Vedic, were transmitted through an unbroken oral tradition for
at least two thousand years before being recorded in the following
texts (these dates are approximate):

- The Vedas, 1500 BCE
- The Upanishads, 800 BCE to 1 CE

- The Bhagavad Gita, 500 BCE
- The Yoga Sutras, 200 BCE*

Vedic philosophers referred to these texts' timeless and universal teachings as *Sanatana Dharma*, which means "Eternal Truth." Sanatana Dharma is an example of spirituality without dogma or the belief that any one group holds exclusive claim to ultimate truth.

One of my favorite teachings of Sanatana Dharma is to believe nothing until you experience it yourself. This path is rooted in direct experience. Yogis are free thinkers, driven to personally explore and realize eternal truths about their true nature and the essence of reality. Sanatana Dharma teaches us how to free ourselves of granthis (knots) in the body and mind so we can experience truth directly. In his book *Introduction to Vedanta*, my grandfather, Narendra Kumar, wrote: "Even a cursory glance of yoga scriptures such as the Vedas and Upanishads reveals that yoga is free from dogma or doctrine. Yoga scriptures free the mind from blind faith and prepare us to discover truth in our own being."

Another defining feature of Sanatana Dharma is its inclusivity and acceptance of different paths. A well-known Vedic hymn beautifully describes this: "As different streams having their sources in different places, all mingle their water in the sea, so different paths people take through different tendencies, various though they appear, all lead to the same truth" (Rigveda 1.164).

According to Sanatana Dharma, the search for truth is deeply personal. Whether one finds it in God, gods, or a godless intellectual is private. Yoga does not require changing your religion, quitting

---

*   Although the Yoga Sutras of Patanjali are not directly a part of Advaita Vedanta, they share the same philosophical commonalities and are seen as complementary. Scholars and practitioners often integrate practices of the Yoga Sutras within the framework of Advaita Vedanta.

your job, or leaving your family. For thousands of years, yoga has been a householder's path. It is a journey of self-realization open to people of all backgrounds, faiths, and walks of life.

एकं सद् विप्राः बहुधा वदन्ति

Ekam sat vipra bahudha vadanti

Truth is one. People call it by various names.

RIGVEDA (1.164.46)

Having a teacher to guide you in your yoga practices is a blessing. A teacher can help you practice most effectively, tailoring each exercise to the state of your mind, body, and spirit. As blocks in the mind and body open, practitioners enjoy a direct, personal, and intimate connection to truth, without any intermediary.

Expansion

The primary purpose of yoga is to know who you are at the level of your soul, and to feel a connection with all life, including Source itself — whether you call it the Universe, the Divine, God, higher power, or something else. For a yogi, the label we place on this mystery isn't what matters. What matters is opening ourself up to have our own experience of it, not as a momentary miracle but as a natural part of daily life. This union can unleash a profound sense of love that can be deeply healing, often transcending scientific and conventional medical understanding.

Another effect of this union is the emergence of *siddhis*, a Sanskrit term for extraordinary abilities such as healing the sick, diagnosing illness, telepathy, and clairvoyance (or remote viewing). These phenomena are not considered exotic. They are available to those who dedicate themselves to meditative disciplines.

There is substantial clinical evidence that various forms of extrasensory perception (ESP) — including clairvoyance, telepathy, and precognition — have operated in daily life since the Stone Age. Historical and contemporary testimonies reveal that clairvoyance is "a latent human capacity." The US government has invested billions of dollars in research on remote viewing, telepathy, precognition, and other psychic abilities, both for intelligence gathering and in broader investigations into human consciousness and perception.

How far have we come in realizing our mind's potential? What will happen when we ignite the full power of our own minds?

Whether you wish to embark on this path to free yourself of kleshas and experience inner peace and/or to explore the full potential of the human mind, this book offers foundational teachings to unlock the mind's power.

Foundations, Pillars, and Principles of the Yogi's Way

There are many methods and schools of thought within yoga traditions. The Yogi's Way is rooted in the ancient Vedic wisdom of yoga and Ayurveda, much of which is now being supported by cutting-edge scientific research. The purpose of this method is to integrate yogic wisdom into the realities of our modern lives, using it to cultivate a mind that leads us to greater peace, creativity, integrity, vitality, and purpose. Through a combination of wisdom and practical techniques, we can dissolve granthis and unlock the pure potential and creative energy within our innermost being.

Four Foundations

A house built on a weak foundation will fall. No matter how beautiful the things we place inside the house are, they don't matter if the house can crumble at any moment. By contrast, when the base is solid, we can flourish.

The four foundations of the Yogi's Way are:

1. **Motivation:** Continually root yourself in the intention to practice for the benefit of all. Commit to discovering, updating, or refining your contribution. What do you want to give?
2. **Stories:** The way you define yourself can bind or liberate you. Create an empowering story.
3. **Choices:** Make decisions that help instead of harm you. Once you realize the power of your thoughts and that you have the capacity to change the ways you think, speak, and act, you are empowered to make better choices.
4. **Nourishment:** Immerse yourself in movement, breath, rest, awareness, and community. Cultivate a healthy lifestyle and make life a celebration.

Twelve Pillars

Pillars provide the support that upholds us and allows us to live with integrity. If even one pillar is unstable, it impacts the entire structure. This is why practicing all twelve pillars is essential.

The twelve pillars of the Yogi's Way are:

1. **Mitras:** Connect with people who support and inspire you.
2. **Breath:** Expand your energy.
3. **Healthy thoughts:** Transform destructive patterns.
4. **Mantra:** Protect your mind.
5. **Visualization:** Believe it to see it.
6. **Meditation:** Develop concentration, stability, and clarity.
7. **Movement:** Release trauma and blocked energy.
8. **Rest:** Restore and renew.

9. **Journaling:** Bring forth what is within you.
10. **Communication:** With love, be transparent.
11. **Nutrition:** Enjoy healthy, delicious food.
12. **Service:** Give without expectation.

Core Principles

At the heart of this method lies a commitment to timeless Vedic wisdom and practical guidance. These are the core principles of the Yogi's Way:

1. Our thoughts, words, and actions shape our reality.
2. Kleshas ravage our health, relationships, and the possibilities of knowing and honoring our svadharma.
3. Every harmful tendency of the mind can be changed.
4. The stories we tell ourselves about who we are have immense power over our lives.
5. The words we use create strongholds in the mind that are hard to dissolve. We must watch our words.
6. Our mind affects the health of our body and the quality of our connection to Spirit. At the root of mind/body/spirit is the mind.
7. The mind can be either a gateway to higher states of consciousness, where we experience expanding states of creativity, joy, peace, and freedom, or a prison that drains our energy, leaving us sick, stuck, and exhausted.
8. In each moment, we have a choice of what we think, say, and do.
9. Who and what we allow into our lives through our senses — what we eat, watch, listen to, see, read — have a huge influence on the mind and on what we do, think, and say. *Guard your gates. Protect your energy.*
10. Knowing our true Self and being rooted in this experience

creates a reliable ground in a confusing, difficult, and uncertain world.

11. Genuine happiness comes from awakening dormant creative energies within ourselves and giving ourselves *to* the world rather than getting things *from* the world. Honor the creative principle within.

12. We rejoice in our practices. Each day, our thoughts, words, and actions align more closely with our deepest wisdom and desires.

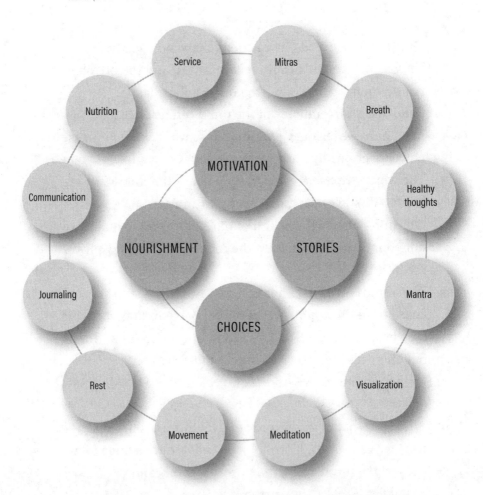

FIGURE 2: The Yogi's Way foundations and pillars.

How to Use This Book

This book is designed as a twelve-week self-guided course. The twelve chapters in the book are written as weeks. Each week, we complete the reading and exercises in one chapter.* The practices at the end of each chapter offer a way for the philosophy to come to life for the reader.

The time commitment for this program includes approximately three hours a week to complete the practices and assignments found at the end of each chapter. In addition, you will gradually build a personal practice. Each week introduces new practice elements that build upon those from previous weeks, culminating in the Yogi's Way Heal Yourself Now® sequence, which you'll find at the end of Week Twelve.

You will want to set aside time for a one-hour weekly meeting with your *mitras*. The concept of mitra — a friend who protects you from harm — is explained in detail in Week One. The meetings can take place in person, over the phone, or online. If you need help finding a mitra, join the Yogi's Way online community (The YogisWay.com/thebook). Here, you may find other practitioners looking to connect and share this twelve-week journey.

As for materials, you will require very little: a pen, a journal, and a quiet, clean space in your home. The space doesn't have to be anything fancy. It can be at the foot of your bed or in a corner of your room. What's important is the intention to keep the space clean — a reflection of the mental, emotional, and physical space you are cultivating within. Just like in a garden, the experience will be much nicer when someone has pulled the weeds, watered the plants, and made it look pleasant. Ideally, the space is simple and comfortable, not too hot or cold, with natural light and fresh air. You will also

---

*   Structuring the book around weeks instead of chapters was inspired by Julia Cameron's seminal 1992 book, *The Artist's Way.*

need a pillow, cushion, or chair to sit on for your meditation and breathing practices and a yoga mat or rug for your movement practices.

Thank you for being here. Blessings on your journey.

Key Terms from the Introduction

Yoga: Union with the true Self.

Mind: The storehouse of thoughts and emotions.

Klesha: Mind poison or destructive emotion.

Body: The complete entity, composed of five layers: physical, energetic, mental, conscious, bliss.

Granthi: Knot or block.

Atman: The true Self, soul, or innermost being.

Svadharma: The right action for you; your role in the cosmic order.

WEEK ONE

MITRAS

Cultivate Friendship and Community

ॐ सह नाववतु।
सह नौ भुनक्तु।
सह वीर्यं करवावहै।
तेजस्वि नावधीतमस्तु मा विद्विषावहै।
ॐ शान्तिः शान्तिः शान्तिः ॥

Om saha navavatu
saha nau bhunaktu
saha viryam karavavahai
tejasvi navadhitamastu ma vidvishavahai
Om shantih, shantih, shantih

Protect us together. Nourish us together.
May our knowledge and strength ever increase.
May we never misunderstand one another.
Om peace, peace, peace.

YAJURVEDA TAITTIRIYA UPANISHAD (2.2)

Call it a clan, call it a network, call it a tribe, call it a family.
Whatever you call it, whoever you are, you need one.
You need one because you are human.

JANE HOWARD, *Families*

The Tibetan master Gyumed Khensur Rinpoche once demonstrated the power of engaging in spiritual practice with friends and community. He held up a pencil, symbolizing the power of practicing alone. With ease, he broke the pencil in half. Then, he held up a handful of pencils, representing the power of practicing in a group. He tried with all his strength but could not break those pencils.

We are stronger together. Alone, we can survive. But together, we create a network of strength, resilience, and support.

Traditionally, yoga was taught in a community setting, which provided an outlet for practitioners to share experiences, ask questions, exchange insights, debate ideas, and cultivate invaluable bonds. In ancient India, there were schools of yoga called *gurukuls*, where one of the requirements was that students have questioning and curious minds. Yoga training included proficiency in debate and critical thinking, ensuring a lively environment with continuous exploration and discovery.

With community, we have opportunities to integrate and understand what we experience in our practices. We share food, music, laughter, service-oriented projects, and heartfelt conversations, which enable us to connect on a deep level. As we ask questions and explore different viewpoints, we develop empathy and the ability to understand various perspectives. We build camaraderie. Doors open. Our journey becomes one of meaningful connections, which often turn into lifelong relationships.

In today's increasingly isolated world, being part of a community is more important than ever. In May 2023, US Surgeon General Dr. Vivek Murthy issued an advisory highlighting our "epidemic of loneliness and isolation," describing it as an underappreciated public health crisis that has significantly hurt individual and societal well-being. His research revealed that at any given moment, about one out of every two Americans experiences measurable levels of loneliness. Murthy noted that social disconnection dramatically increases the risk of anxiety and depression, often doubling it. He emphasized that "rebuilding social connection must be a top public health priority for our nation" and advocated creating programs that foster human connection, comparing our need for social bonds to our need for food and water.

In 2006, while living in New York City, I was part of a dynamic community of yogis. We practiced every morning for ninety minutes. Our practice consisted of mantra, pranayama, asana (the physical postures), philosophy, meditation, and deep relaxation. Often, we would meet in the evenings and discuss our practices while sharing a nutritious meal. On weekends, we attended workshops and trainings through which we deepened our knowledge and strength, just as the mantra at the top of this chapter encourages us to do. We didn't always open up about the most personal challenges we were going through, but we had one thing in common: We were transforming our minds, bodies, health, and lives. While meeting consistently, we deeply bonded in this experience.

Community gives us momentum to keep up with our practices. When we are feeling tired, down, or unmotivated, our friends and community inspire us to take the time we need to rest and be alone while also encouraging us to get back up. Without this support, we risk embarking on a downward spiral and sinking into old patterns.

The support we receive from community is especially important today as we are so easily distracted by our handheld devices and additional electronics offering endless streams of entertainment and other consumables. Big tech has invested billions of dollars in developing these platforms to dominate our attention and influence our thoughts, choices, and actions. Through yoga, we cultivate discipline, focus, and the ability to choose what we pay attention to. Developing these skills alongside mitras and in community enriches the journey and makes it enduring.

Mitra: A Friend Who Protects You from Harm

A cornerstone of the Yogi's Way is maintaining weekly connections with a group of two to three mitras.

The Sanskrit word *mitra* translates as "friend." It is a combination of the root words *mi*, which means "destruction," and *tra*, meaning "protective force." Your mitras are friends who protect you from harm — not just the dangers of the world, but the ways that we harm ourselves through our own choices, words, actions, and thoughts.

In the Vedas, Mitra is a deity who symbolizes honesty, friendship, contracts, and meetings. In Zoroastrianism, Mithra is the protector and keeper of truth, friendship, promises, and love. In Tibetan Buddhism, Maitreya is the bodhisattva known to be kind and loving.

Mitras listen to us with compassion. They hold us accountable with love. They help us become aware of the ways in which we limit ourselves. Mitras support us to move through our kleshas and experience higher states of consciousness. So often, our friends can see in us what we cannot.

Our mitras become our accountability partners. Without accountability, we often fail to practice consistently, and consistency is necessary for growth. The American Society of Training and Development found that people who have an accountability partner are 65 percent more likely to reach their goals. For those who set up regular check-ins with their partner, the percentage skyrockets to 95 percent. When we have someone to be accountable to and to share our experiences with, we are much more likely to stay motivated and to keep our commitments.

Research from the *Journal of Clinical Psychology* indicates that about 54 percent of people who attempt to shift their habits fail to sustain the transformation longer than six months. On average, individuals attempt the same personal goal ten times without success. According to this research, the challenge isn't knowing what to do but committing to the change. The Yogi's Way mitra practice was designed to support individuals in making lasting transformations.

There is a humility in journeying together on a spiritual path. We have the privilege of witnessing our mitras' process and connecting deeper with our own. No matter how much self-work we have partaken of, our human nature is to evolve. There is no end to how much we can heal, expand, and deepen.

In her research on the science of happiness, Dr. Sonja Lyubomirsky of the University of California, Riverside, found that those who engaged in acts of kindness toward themselves were happy in the moment, but the happiness did not last. Those who engaged in acts of kindness toward others became happier and stayed happier for two to four weeks. Our mitras provide us this opportunity.

With our mitras, we practice vulnerability and courage. Clarity is born from these exchanges. As we journey to the center of our being, we simultaneously cultivate a connection with the creative forces of the Universe. As doors to our soul open inwardly, doors also open outwardly.

Several years ago, two of my good friends, Emily and Anita, had never met and didn't even know about each other. They'd separately shared with me that they were struggling in their own ways. I had a strong feeling that I had to create a circumstance where the three of us would build an alliance and help one another. I contacted them separately and explained my thoughts. We agreed to a group call, and I scheduled a Zoom session, as we were scattered across the US. I presented them with an idea to set up a twelve-week study group to go through a specific set of yoga practices together. It was structured with daily practices, journaling, and awareness exercises as well as with weekly calls to discuss thoughts, questions, blocks, and breakthroughs. They enthusiastically agreed to try it.

What happened in those twelve weeks for each of us was mind-blowing. In the past, I had done these same yoga practices alone. The dramatic difference of practicing with my mitras was one of the most powerful experiences of my life. We *became* those pencils that Rinpoche spoke about. Our connection, intention, and commitment created an otherworldly space where magic unfolded. As the weeks passed, we were sending one another quotes, inspiring one another with the small changes we were making in our daily lives, and shifting our own realities. Two of us helped the other get out of a long-term abusive relationship. Another helped one of us refine our most treasured gift and actually start sharing it with our community. Another one got her dream job after becoming crystal clear on exactly what she wanted. All of this happened in twelve weeks with three mitras.

That process changed each of our lives and inspired the mitra practice that is the first pillar of the Yogi's Way. Over the years, I've witnessed many lives completely transform through such shared experience. Our inner circle is worth its weight in gold.

Week One Practices

1. *Choose Your Mitras*

Engaging your yoga journey with the support of mitras helps you overcome the kleshas of loneliness and isolation, which have become epidemics in our modern world and can lead to mental and physical unrest. To begin the process of choosing your mitras, identify the people in your life who influence you in positive or negative ways. They may be colleagues, friends, family members, authors, artists, contacts on social media, people you know well, or people you haven't personally met. Some of them may not be alive, and that's OK — you may include them too.

In your notebook, make a two-circle Venn diagram like the one shown in figure 3. In the first circle, list the people who discourage or distract you from taking time for yourself. Consider for each one: Is this a toxic relationship? Do you enable them to distract you? Are you subconsciously blocking yourself by having this person in your life?

For the second circle, think of the people who are your champions, who encourage and love you for who you are. Write down those names here.

As you fill in both circles, you may realize that life is often not that black-and-white. In the overlapping section, write down the names of those who play both roles.

Figure 3 shows the overlap possible between these groups.

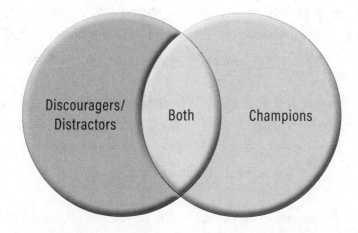

FIGURE 3: Distractors, champions, and those who are both.

Look at your list of champions and pick one or two people who are alive now, whom you have contact with, and who you feel are solid and reliable friends — not part of a codependent relationship but part of one that is rooted in mutual care. In the next twenty-four hours, reach out to these friends. Explain to them what a mitra signifies. Tell them that you are embarking on a twelve-week journey to transform your mind, health, and reality so that you can experience your full potential. Ask them to join you. The commitment is a one-hour weekly meeting with your mitras on the phone, online, or in person. Approximately one hour of daily practice is also included in your commitments.

If you can't find a mitra, dig deeper. Perhaps your mitra is a colleague you haven't spoken to in years, a childhood friend you could reconnect with, or a person in your community, family, work, or friend circle whom you aren't close with but have always felt a kinship toward.

You can also reach out to the Yogi's Way online community, where you may find like-minded people looking to connect with mitras. In addition, the Yogi's Way offers live twelve-week programs (online or in person) where you are paired with mitras through a real-time collective experience. If you choose this option, still move forward with this book. Going through it on your own is a great way to prepare for a live experience.

To connect with the Yogi's Way community and see upcoming online and in-person events, visit TheYogisWay.com/thebook.

2. Find Your Motivation

Yoga helps us minimize kleshas and experience the highest reality.

Yoga Sutras (2.2)

*We conquer every struggle within the mind
to be united with the love in all.*

Taittiriya Upanishad (3.10.3–4)

At the heart of The Yogi's Way is the process of working through our kleshas so we can experience higher states of consciousness, enabling us to live up to our greatest potential. But healing is not a linear journey. In this course, some days you will feel like you're making profound breakthroughs, and some days you will feel like you're walking through mud. That's why it's important to establish a clear motivation as to why you want to embark on this path. Your motivation and your mitras will help you stick with your practices.

To practice yoga for self-gratification doesn't get us far on the path. When our motivation is to awaken blocked energy so we can give to the world (instead of get from the world), we come into a powerful alignment that supports our practice. One of India's great yogis, Sri Nisargadatta Maharaj, said: "Desire the good of all and the universe will work with you."

Why do you want to overcome kleshas and unite with the light and potential that live within? In your own words, write down your motivation in a couple of sentences. Once you write down your motivation, place it where you will see it every day — a sticky note on your bathroom mirror, at the very front of your journal or laptop, or by your bedside table. Read it every day as you move through this course and let it inspire you.

When we begin to live for a higher purpose than ourselves,
an intense fire is ignited deep in our consciousness,
inflaming our enthusiasm and determination.

Eknath Easwaran

When I was struggling most with kleshas, I realized that my three-year-old daughter was watching me and absorbing everything I was experiencing. On *Oprah's Super Soul* podcast, I heard the great psychotherapist Dr. Edith Eva Eger say, "Children don't do what we say. They do what they see." At that moment, my daughter became my motivation. I wanted to get myself out of a dark and limited place in my mind *for her*. I wanted her to know that our wounds can be opportunities to dig deeper into the resources that lie within us and that make life meaningful, purposeful, and genuinely joyful.

I wanted to unearth those treasures within myself and fill our lives with purpose, creativity, and fun. Kids know what's genuine and what's a show. Dr. Eger was right. It doesn't matter what we say to our children. It matters what they see us do. If we adults learn to work through our kleshas and ignite the power of our minds, we can be an example for the next generation.

Your motivation can be something simple, like, "I want to live to my full potential." Or "I want to contribute my gifts to my greatest capacity." When Sonia, a student in our community, did this course, she realized that her motivation wasn't exactly external. Her motivation was "mental clarity" so she could extend her energy into helping her community instead of engaging in negative mental play.

Enjoy finding your own expression of what motivates you.

3. Journey Inward: Self-Healing versus Selfishness

Only a few are wise enough to turn their gaze inwards.

KATHA UPANISHAD (2.1.1)

It is important to dedicate time every day to our journey inward. To reserve such space in your life requires an understanding that it is not selfish to engage in the deep work of healing ourselves. We have to take care of ourselves to have energy and authenticity for the world. Vedic texts emphasize selflessness as an integral part of the path. It is essential that this not be misunderstood. We are here, all of us interconnected. Perhaps the very purpose of life is to care for the life around us, whether that is our children, friends, family, pets, or nature. *We must recognize ourselves as a part of this equation.* It is an absolute must to prioritize our own care, every single day. Not to do so is not a minor neglect. It is *dangerous.* In the words of the physician and bestselling author Dr. Gabor Maté: "The need to please people all the time will kill you."

In his book *When the Body Says No*, Dr. Maté addresses the mind-body connection. Based in Canada, while researching and treating people with such chronic illnesses as cancer and autoimmune diseases, he found that even though conventional medical science says we don't know why these diseases come about, the reasons are actually clear. Dr. Maté found striking similarities in patterns of behavior and personality traits in those who suffered from cancer and autoimmune diseases. They were givers, so dedicated to their families, communities, and jobs that they never took a day off, even when they were in great pain. They never asked for help. They were so "kind" and agreeable that they didn't show anger or sadness. In other words, they repressed their emotions, ignored their own needs, and were not true to themselves.

"The automatic and compulsive concern for the needs of others while ignoring your own is a major risk factor for chronic illness," Maté says. It is not the patient's fault, he explains. They aren't aware of what they are doing. If you identify with the role of the pleaser who neglects their own needs, it is not your fault either. We all carry roles, whether it is a result of our culture, society, history, or family dynamics. Many of us didn't learn how to say no. We were socialized to say yes even when we didn't mean it. It requires a huge rewiring of the brain to change this.

In Ayurveda, the medical side of yoga, repressing emotions is recognized as one of the root causes of illness. Now, through extensive research and case studies, science has confirmed that repressing emotions such as anger suppresses the immune system. According to Dr. Maté, when a person isn't true to themselves, emotions get confused. Then the immune system gets confused, and it turns against itself. Autoimmune illnesses result. Again, this is not the patient's fault. This is how many of us were programmed, especially women. It is no surprise that 80 percent of the people with autoimmune disease are women. Women are acculturated to play a certain role: to be responsible for people's emotions, suppress healthy anger, absorb the stresses of the family, and not disappoint. Maté says: "If you don't know how to say no, the body will do it for you in the form of illness."

4. Establish Boundaries

On this path, while you are carving out time for your daily practices, creating boundaries becomes important. We only have so many breaths in this life. Start saying no when your body says no, not out of malice for anyone, but out of love for yourself. Say yes to yourself out of wisdom, knowing that your health and integrity are the foundation for you to give in ways that are most effective and meaningful. Remember, our motivation to practice is to have more energy and wisdom to give. However, if we give without caring for ourselves, we will fall.

When you start saying no, if guilt arises, be with the guilt. See that part of yourself. Don't turn away from it or judge it. Instead, turn toward it. Accept it. Tell that part of yourself that you are here to listen to what it has to say. With compassion and love, listen to the part of you that feels guilty. Thank it for trying to protect you and care for you in its own way. Then, ask it if it would please step aside and allow you to care for yourself.

Change is hard, and it takes time, but this is how we begin to heal not just ourselves but generations before and after us.

In what areas of your life are you saying yes when your truth is no? Work? Relationships? Write them down in your journal. What we track, we can monitor. What we monitor, we can begin to recognize as patterns. With awareness, we can begin to change harmful patterns.

What shifts can you start to make in your life now to build up to carving out one hour every day for your inner journey? Next week, you will begin a ten- to fifteen-minute daily practice. In Week

Three, that will turn into thirty-five to forty-five minutes. By Week Eight, you will have a forty- to fifty-five-minute daily practice. Start to prepare now to create this time for yourself by setting healthy boundaries around your schedule. The best time for practice is early morning, after a beverage and shower, or early evening,.

5. Seek Blessings

Ancient civilizations throughout the world have had practices to offer respect to and ask for blessings from elders. Call to mind a few people whom you admire most: ancestors, guides, guardians, colleagues, friends, neighbors — anyone. It's OK if they've passed away or are alive, if you've met them personally or not. From a quiet place in your heart, call these beings to your mind. Tell them that you are embarking on a journey of healing and awakening so that you have more energy to give. Ask them to bless your journey, especially as it entails facing every obstacle in the mind. Ask with sincerity and earnestness. Visualize them one by one. Take your time with each being. Then, feel their blessings pour upon you like the most refreshing rain or the sweetest sunlight. See yourself and your journey as blessed. Give thanks and ask them to please stay close in the space of your heart.

My grandmother's favorite mantra carries the feeling of this exercise. It is called "Prabhujee."* Here's the translation of this mantra:

> Divine being, have compassion for me. Come, reside in my heart.
> Without you, I feel a hollowness inside. Fill up my bare entity with love.

---

* You can hear a recording of the song "Prabhujee" on *Truth Love Creation*, my first mantra album, released by Nettwerk Music and streaming on all major platforms.

I don't know the rituals, chants, and prayers. I just know that I
believe in you.
I searched the whole world for you. Now, please come, take my
hand, and guide me.

If this practice feels uncomfortable to you or you can't think of
anyone to call on, imagine the highest version of yourself. Visualize
the qualities of this being. Invite this person into your heart. Ask
them to remain close.

Week One Mitra Meeting

Set a time for your weekly mitra meeting. This is a very special and
sacred window of time you are carving out to honor your potential and purpose. It's best to keep your meetings to the same day
and time each week for this twelve-week course. Each mitra will
take turns leading the weekly meetings. With your mitras, decide
who will lead the first one. Allow each mitra time to share as much
of their week's experiences as they feel comfortable. How does it
feel to begin this journey? To write down your motivation, establish
boundaries, and ask for blessings? Share as much of your experience
and answers as you like. Are there any teachings covered so far that
you'd all like to debate and discuss — for example, the definition of
yoga offered in the introduction?

Start and end your weekly mitra meetings with the mantra at the
beginning of this chapter (page 17). Recite the English translation
together with your mitras to set the tone for a powerful experience.
"Protect us together. Nourish us together. May our knowledge and
strength ever increase. May we never misunderstand one another.
Om peace, peace, peace." Try chanting the Sanskrit version if you'd
like. For support, you can listen to a recording of the Sanskrit at
TheYogisWay.com/thebook.

Key Terms from Week One

Mitra: A friend who protects you from harm, with whom you form an alliance and bond. Derived from the Vedic deity Mitra, who is prominent in the Rigveda and is the patron of honesty, friendship, promises, and agreements.

Asana: Physical postures.

Pranayama: Breathing practices.

KLESHAS

Identify Harmful Thoughts and Emotions

*There is no greater victory in the life of a human being
than victory over the mind...the true soldier is the one who
fights not the external but the internal foes.*

SWAMI RAMDAS

*"What's the bravest thing you've ever said?" asked the boy.
"Help," said the horse.*

CHARLIE MACKESY, *The Boy, the Mole, the Fox, and the Horse*

The wisdom of the earliest yoga texts recognizes that the most important battles we will face in our lives are within ourselves — our own anger, attachment, fear, jealousy, and anxiety.*

One of the most beloved texts of yogic wisdom, the Bhagavad Gita, is an epic conversation between two mitras. The story sheds light on the harmful tendencies of the mind and how we can overcome them. In the beginning of the story, one of the friends, Arjuna, is overwhelmed with kleshas and in a state of despair. Arjuna is the greatest warrior of the land and renowned for his bravery. Yet he finds himself afflicted with so much anxiety, sorrow, self-pity,

---

* These texts include the Vedas, Upanishads, Bhagavad Gita, and Yoga Sutras.

confusion, and shame that he is sweating and shaking, with eyes full of tears. His bow slips from his hand, and he falls to the ground, unable to get up.

Arjuna has a decision to make that affects all those he loves. He is unclear about his svadharma — the right action for him. In a moment of complete humility and desperation, he turns to Krishna and asks for help. "I have no idea what to do," Arjuna confides in his friend.

There's no shame in admitting that we experience any of the kleshas. In fact, acknowledging that we have kleshas is the first step to freeing ourselves from them.

Each and every detail in the Bhagavad Gita, a work approximately a thousand pages long, is of monumental significance in helping us understand the war that rages within our minds. People spend a lifetime studying this text, which is filled with such depth of meaning that each time you read it, you experience deeper realizations. Here, I offer a succinct summary of the story.

The setting: Arjuna and Krishna are in a chariot at the center of a battlefield, on the brink of war. Both sides are braced to fight. In the midst of heat, noise, and thousands of people eagerly waiting for Arjuna to make the first move, Arjuna shares his confusion and mental unrest with Krishna. Even in this charged and chaotic moment, Krishna possesses a clear and relaxed mind. He is able to pause, go inward, and then ask his mitra to do the same. Nothing is more important to Krishna than helping his friend understand and overcome the turmoil in his mind. The moment to do it is *now*. Everything else can wait. No matter how much time it takes (which ends up being a lot), Krishna is dedicated to helping Arjuna come to clarity and peace.

Krishna's first instruction to Arjuna is "Behold the *Kurus*." The term *Kurus* refers to the warriors on both sides of the battlefield. On one side stand hundreds of warriors driven by anger, greed,

arrogance, envy, and lies. On the other side, there are only five warriors, and they embody empathy, kindness, generosity, humility,
and love. This imagery is a metaphor for the human mind: We often
wrestle with hundreds of destructive thoughts while only a few nurturing ones arise.

The spiritual journey begins with the most basic and essential
step — "Behold the Kurus" — meaning: Behold your mind. Observe
the full spectrum of your thoughts and emotions — the pleasant,
the painful, and everything in between. Whereas the mind tends to
resist pain and grasp pleasure, allow yourself to be fully present with
all that arises within you. Whether it's anxiety, anger, empathy, or
love, approach these states with nonjudgment and curiosity.

As you take this inward journey, be in touch with your heart-
breaks as well as your joys. Understand your weaknesses as well
as your strengths. Recognize what it is within you that hurts you
and others and what aspects within you are a gift. Be aware of what
thoughts you are having and what choices you are making that give
rise to a mind that either binds you or propels you to expand into
your true potential.

In this way, Krishna sets up the path of yoga. Once we are able
to objectively see what's happening within us, we can begin the
spiritual journey to overcome the destructive tendencies within
ourselves — that is, our kleshas. As pathways clear, dormant and
blocked energies awaken. We get to know who we are beyond our
ever-changing parade of thoughts, emotions, sensations, and experiences.

With Krishna by his side, Arjuna chooses the difficult path
to face his wounds (kleshas) and clear the blocks (granthis) he is
carrying within. During the rest of this epic story, Krishna and
Arjuna share a remarkable inner journey, confronting Arjuna's kleshas with wisdom, tenderness, and affection. Arjuna doesn't blindly
believe what Krishna says. Instead, he asks question after question.

The two friends debate philosophies and ideas around meditation, detachment, service, and the immortal soul.

During their epic conversation, Krishna doesn't tell Arjuna what decision to make. However, by the end of the story, after all the wisdom and practices are exchanged, Arjuna has cleared his blocks and opened pathways to his own innate wisdom. Without a doubt, Arjuna knows what to do. He makes his decision and confidently walks his path with his body and mind strong, focused, and purposeful.

We practice yoga to learn to do what Arjuna did: to work through our kleshas with love, understanding, and support, ultimately to transform our mind from one that is anxious and confused to one that is clear and firm.

The psychospiritual teachings of Carl Jung and the works of Mahatma Gandhi, Martin Luther King Jr., Annie Besant, Ralph Waldo Emerson, Nikola Tesla, and Rukmini Devi Arundale were greatly influenced by the Bhagavad Gita. In his masterpiece, *Walden*, Henry David Thoreau wrote, "In the morning I bathe my intellect in the stupendous and cosmogonal philosophy of the Bhagvat Geeta." Any human who has suffered has gleaned invaluable inspiration as they studied this profound text.

Kleshas: Mind Poisons, Destructive Emotions

Klesha (क्लेश) is a Sanskrit word that translates to "mind poison" or "destructive emotion." The Yoga Sutras describe kleshas as obstacles to spiritual growth and the cause of suffering. The text identifies the five major kleshas as delusion, attachment, anger, pride, and fear. The Yogi's Way also addresses the kleshas of shame, depression, anxiety, loneliness, and jealousy, because of their prevalence in our world today.

In the Bhagavad Gita, Krishna reveals that he is not merely a friend to Arjuna, but a divine being filled with immeasurable light and wisdom, meant to help and uplift others. Krishna teaches Arjuna — and all of us — that we carry this same light within, along with the potential to be a blessing to those around us. Through the practices of yoga, which include self-reflection and contemplative techniques, we unlock our inner light. This requires us to acknowledge and delve into the roots of our wounds.

In contemporary yoga and spiritual settings, we speak about "letting go" of uncomfortable thoughts and emotions. Devi, a yogini (female yogi) living in the forests of North India who was encountered by author Daniel Odier, warned that if we let go too soon — before we experience an emotion fully — we imprison ourselves, because the wound isn't healed. It either lingers on or comes back with greater force. She said, "Everybody wants to let go. But how do you let go if you don't hold things, if you don't touch things in full consciousness, with a totally open heart? If you let go before touching deeply that can bring on severe mental turmoil. Many beginning yogis make this mistake."

The Yogi's Way addresses the kleshas described below. Keep in mind that kleshas are not inherently "good" or "bad." They are a part of the human experience and carry important messages for us to receive. On this path, we learn to acknowledge our kleshas and move through them in constructive ways. This frees us of the damaging grip they can have on us — a theme explored throughout this book.

Delusion, confusion (अविद्या *avidya*): Literal translation is "not wisdom." It refers to a false idea of reality or mistaking illusion for reality — for example, seeing the impermanent as permanent or not understanding that the true Self is full of potential and interconnected with all life. *Avidya* is considered the root cause of all other kleshas.

Attachment (राग *ragah*):* Refers to the attachment to pleasurable experiences. Pleasure itself is not a poison, but chasing, grasping, and clinging to it is. We can get attached to instant gratification instead of what truly benefits us and others in the long term. This can lead to substance abuse and addiction. We may become attached to the outcome of our actions instead of fully engaging with the present moment. Attachments can manifest in various forms — whether to a person, event, job, house, or relationship having to be a certain way. One of the most significant attachments is to our own identity, which can create immense stress and limitation. This will be explored further in "Week Five: Stories."

Anger (द्वेष *dvesha*): *Dvesha* is translated as "aversion," which often gives rise to anger. It refers to a strong feeling of annoyance, displeasure, dislike, hostility, or repulsion toward things that are difficult or unpleasant. If we avoid what we dislike, we suffer. The opposite of this is acceptance. For example, if we push away anger we are feeling toward a good friend, the anger comes back to us intensified. If we accept the anger, befriend it, and come to understand it, its hold on us lessens. The mind may open to insight on how to approach our friend and have a meaningful and calm discussion about what has upset us.

Isolation, loneliness (अस्मिता *asmita*): In the Yoga Sutras, *asmita* is translated as "pride" or "ego." It is characterized by falsely identifying with the ego, which leads to a sense of disconnection from one's true nature. Recognizing the "epidemic of loneliness and isolation" (as the US surgeon general described it) we are facing today, I am applying the concept of asmita to address isolation and loneliness, which often stem from a sense of pride, ego, and separateness.

---

* The yogic definition of attachment is different from attachment theories in the field of psychotherapy.

Fear (अभिनिवेशः *abhinivesha*): In the original texts, *abhinivesha* is explained as "fear, especially of death," or the instinct to protect the physical body. In *The Yogi's Way*, we expand this definition to include the fear of loss, low finances, and uncertainty.

Jealousy (ईर्ष्या *irshya*): A state of feeling envious or covetous; being unable to bear the accomplishments or good fortunes of others. The antidote for jealousy is to rejoice for others' fortunes and blessings. In this moment, you can take a couple of deep breaths and see how it feels in your body to feel jealousy toward someone. Now, close your eyes, breathe deeply, and explore how it feels to rejoice for another's happiness. Kleshas often take weeks and months to transform — but sometimes, transformation can happen in a moment.

Shame (शर्म *sharm*): A painful feeling of humiliation or distress. Shame researcher Dr. Brené Brown defines it as "the intensely painful feeling or experience of believing that we are flawed and therefore unworthy of love and belonging — something we've experienced, done, or failed to do makes us unworthy of connection." Week Six is dedicated to addressing and working through this klesha.

Depression, sorrow (दुःख *dukkha*): a condition characterized by persistent feelings of sadness, hopelessness, and a lack of interest in activities that were once enjoyable. Common symptoms of depression also include a change in appetite, difficulty sleeping or sleeping too much, fatigue, feelings of worthlessness, difficulty concentrating and making decisions, and suicidal ideation. Major depressive disorder is the leading cause of disability in the US for ages fifteen to forty-four. In 2020, over 37 million Americans took antidepressants.

Anxiety (चिन्ताशून्यम् *chintashoonyam*): A feeling of worry, nervousness, or unease, typically about an imminent event or something with an uncertain outcome. Anxiety disorders are the most common mental illness in the US, affecting about 40 million adults ages eighteen and older, or approximately 18.1 percent of the population, every year. The World Health Organization stated in 2019 that 301 million people suffer from anxiety disorders globally.

If you resonate with any of these kleshas — or most of them — *you are not alone.* Allow an awareness of your kleshas to foster a sense of unity with humanity, generating both humility toward yourself and compassion for others. As mentioned in the introduction, I've personally navigated through all the kleshas. To a lesser degree, I still do. Uncomfortable emotions will always come and go. The key lies in embracing their presence without judgment, acknowledging them as an integral part of our human experience. By accepting our humanness and the full spectrum of emotion, we diminish the intensity of kleshas. As a result, they exert less influence over us, allowing us to observe their arrival and departure with more equanimity. This frees us to explore the field of consciousness that lies beyond the movements of the mind. You will experience this phenomenon as you move through the teachings and practices in this book.

Throughout my experience in yoga and healing, I haven't encountered a single person who hasn't had personal traumas or struggled with kleshas. Through my own journey and those of many students, I've come to understand that whether we are facing personal, generational, or collective trauma, it *is* possible to heal ourselves. We *can* free ourselves from the grip of kleshas and enjoy a life of expansion — rich with meaningful relations, creativity, purpose, and genuine, lasting peace. What Arjuna did over three thousand years ago — transforming his distressed mind into one that was clear, grounded, and strong — we can do today.

Week Two Practices

1. Recognize Your Kleshas

The wound is the place where the light enters you.

RUMI

In this practice, we begin to meet our kleshas with curiosity and love and with the intention to understand rather than judge. The purpose of this practice is to identify your major kleshas. In your notebook, write your kleshas in numbered order, starting with the most dominant. When you are in the thick of your most difficult moments, what have been the kleshas that were most intense for you? Jealousy? Fear? Depression? Anger?

As outlined above, the kleshas we focus on in the Yogi's Way are delusion or confusion, attachment, anger, isolation or loneliness, fear, jealousy, shame, depression or sorrow, and anxiety. What are your top three?

2. The Klesha Trigger Log: What Triggers Your Kleshas?

Identifying our kleshas is one step toward developing awareness. Recognizing what triggers our kleshas takes our understanding to another level. As we get to know our emotions and what sets us off, we get better at noticing when we are triggered. This prepares us to be able to take a few breaths and respond to the situation from the discerning higher mind instead of reacting from the impulsive lower mind. When we react to a trigger, we usually don't help ourselves or anyone involved. In one moment, we can react in a way that we regret, causing or deepening a wound or even destroying a relationship. As we become familiar with our triggers, we prepare ourselves to be aware *while* a triggering incident is taking place. This helps us to be able to pause and respond with awareness.

A Klesha Trigger Log (KTL)* is a great tool for increasing your awareness of what triggers you. Every time you get triggered this week, write about the event in your journal as soon as possible after it happens. Aim to be aware of the incident while it is happening. Use these questions as prompts to help you notice the subtleties of your experience:

- In your account of the incident, describe what happened, who was involved, and where you were. What thoughts, words, images, sensations, memories, actions, and emotions — including kleshas — were provoked in you?
- Identify what exactly triggered you and how much time it took for you to realize that you were experiencing harmful thoughts and emotions.
- Describe how your body felt when you were provoked. Did your jaw tighten, your brow furrow, your belly squeeze, your shoulders tense, your face heat up, your voice change?
- Did your mind become clouded, affecting your discernment?
- How long did you remain upset?
- How do you feel about the incident now? Is there anything else that could have contributed to it — for example, were you hungry or thirsty? Had you exercised that day or gotten fresh air? Did something happen earlier in the day or week that could have instigated the trigger?
- Having had this moment to reflect on the incident, how would you respond differently if you were in this situation again?

---

*   This practice was inspired by the Cultivating Emotional Balance program run by Dr. Eve Ekman.

Here is an opportunity to practice *intelligent regret*. This is the only useful type of regret, because it doesn't consist of guilt or shame. Instead, you review what happened with a compassionate mind. You recognize how your reaction hurt you or another, and you accept it while deciding not to do it again. As Oprah Winfrey says Maya Angelou once told her, "When you know better, you do better." Instead of shaming yourself, celebrate your growing awareness.

In a moment of total peace, when you are in a calm state, it is possible for you to trigger yourself. Your mind can go to a memory from the past or an imagined scenario about the future and create harmful thoughts and emotions. In this case, a trigger may not be an external event, but something born from the mind while in a quiet space. If you experience this, journal about it while asking yourself the same questions above.

3. Establish Optimal Breathing

The journey to the infinite core of our being is arduous.
Pranic breathing can take us there.

B. K. S. IYENGAR

The foundation of all yoga practices is slow breathing through the nose. Especially as we engage in the courageous and vulnerable inner work this course requires, it is important to stay connected to your breath. This week, we will develop a habit to breathe slowly and deeply through the nose *throughout the day*. We will start by learning how to establish optimal breathing. This type of breathing activates the body's relaxation response. It modulates emotional regions of the brain, helping to relieve emotional distress and tension.

Every morning, after you get ready for your day and before you head out to work, take the kids to school, or start on your day's project, take five minutes to establish optimal breathing.

Five-Minute Optimal Breath Practice

Sit comfortably on the floor or on a chair. If seated on the floor, place a pillow or cushion under the back of the hips to support a straight spine. If seated on a chair, keep both feet flat on the floor. Turn off notifications on your phone and set a timer for five minutes.

Relax your shoulders, hips, and the muscles of your face, especially your jaw. Lengthen your spine by rooting your hips down and gently lifting your heart toward the sky. Keep your shoulders relaxed, drawn down and back, and aligned over the hips, ensuring your posture remains balanced without leaning forward or back.

Bring awareness to your breath. Place one hand on your belly and one hand on your upper chest. Inhale slowly through your nose and feel the belly naturally rise. Exhale through the nose and feel the belly naturally move in toward the spine.

Continue to breathe slowly through the nose. Close the mouth and relax the lips. Let the tip of the tongue rest on the top palate behind the front teeth. Try to keep the chest as still as possible, with only the belly moving.

Relax into a comfortable rhythm of breathing. You can try taking an inhalation and exhalation that are approximately 6 seconds each. In his 2020 book *Breath*, journalist James Nestor reported that contemporary research found a 5.5-second inhalation and 5.5-second exhalation to be optimal. If this feels like a strain or uncomfortable at all, reduce the count as much as you need — to a 2-, 3-, 4-, or 5-second inhale and an equal length of exhale. Relax into a rhythm that feels natural to you. The length of your breath will extend in the coming weeks and months as you practice. Controlling your breath will eventually help you to control your reactions and consciously choose where to place your energy.

4. All-Day Yoga: A New and Powerful Habit

Throughout your day, stay connected to the slow and steady nasal breathing of the five-minute Optimal Breath practice while maintaining the posture you cultivated. I call this ongoing practice All-Day Yoga, or ADY.* This one habit will literally change your life, bringing healing and vital energy to your body and focus and ease to your mind. As you move through your day, be aware not to breathe only into your chest, which amplifies anxiety and the experience of other kleshas. Make sure to drop the breath down to the belly and relax as you breathe deeply and slowly, feeling the belly naturally expand on the inhalations and contract on the exhalations. This will have the immediate effect of relieving the intensity that fear and other kleshas often bring. When you are feeling especially anxious or stressed, make the exhales a little longer than your inhalations. You can lengthen the exhalations to be 1.5 times or two times longer than the inhalations. For example, inhaling for four counts and exhaling for six counts can help calm the mind down.

The quality of our breathing determines the amount of vital energy that moves into the body, oxygenates our cells, and helps us create and maintain a grounded and relaxed foundation. In *Breath*, Nestor wrote that the average person takes about 25,000 breaths in a day. The quality of our breath affects every aspect of our health, from the density of our bones to the subatomic level of our electrons. Scientific research reveals that breathing slowly through the nose transforms our mental and physical health.

Nestor found that nearly 50 percent of people are chronic mouth breathers, a habit that causes chronic stress and exhaustion. When

---

*   I was introduced to this phrase in my studies of Tibetan heart yoga, which is rooted in the Gelukpa tradition, in 2009.

one is breathing through the nose, air is purified, warmed, moistened, and pressurized. Nasal breathing boosts nitric oxide production in the paranasal sinuses sixfold, which facilitates vasodilation, enhances elimination of carbon dioxide, and allows 18 percent more oxygen to be absorbed by the body than through mouth breathing. This helps sustain our energy throughout the day. It leads to mental clarity, lower blood pressure, decreased stress, and increased blood circulation throughout the body. Nestor's research also explained the importance of diaphragmatic breathing, which is a foundational technique in pranayama. This type of breathing uses primarily the diaphragm instead of the chest. It requires less effort and energy while reducing stress and anxiety and improving overall health and wellness.

The benefits of slow, deep nasal breathing on mental and physical health are many:

- It modulates the emotional regions of the brain and relieves emotional distress and tension. Fear, stress, and anxiety change breathing patterns, making them more shallow and rapid.
- It activates the body's relaxation response.
- The nasal passageway warms and humidifies inhaled air, offering protection to the respiratory system.
- It enhances sleep quality, boosts energy levels, and promotes mental clarity.
- It facilitates the release of toxins: Approximately 70 percent of toxins can be expelled through proper breathing techniques.
- It alleviates physical pain.
- It combats allergies.
- It improves digestion.
- It elevates mood.
- It improves oral health by reducing the risk of gingivitis,

periodontitis, receding gums, cavities, oral decay, and halitosis (bad breath).

- It regulates and optimizes the body's oxygen and carbon dioxide levels.
- It offers numerous cardiovascular benefits, including lowering blood pressure, strengthening the immune system, increasing brain function, improving exercise performance, and reducing the risk of erectile dysfunction and other health-related functions associated with blood flow.

Week Two Daily Practice Sequence

1. Every morning, take five minutes to establish slow, deep diaphragmatic breathing through the nose, following the Optimal Breath practice instructions on page 44.
2. Continue this breathing throughout the day for All-Day Yoga.
3. Every evening, spend five to ten minutes on the Klesha Trigger Log.

Total daily practice time: ten to fifteen minutes

Week Two Mitra Meeting

Go to your mitra meeting prepared, with all the practices completed. Remember to take turns each week as the leader of your meetings. That person is responsible for reminding the group of the next meeting, inspiring the group throughout the week by sharing relevant quotes and stories, and knowing the week's chapter inside and out to help lead the group toward understanding.

At the meeting, share how the practices were for you. What is your experience as you begin to explore your kleshas? Any surprises? What have you learned about yourself so far as you keep a

Klesha Trigger Log? How does it feel to breathe deeply through the nose throughout the day?

If you feel uncomfortable sharing your experiences, remind yourself and your team that all the information shared in your meetings is private and doesn't leave the trusted circle you are cultivating. Sharing so intimately may not be easy, but we experience insight and growth when we stretch out of our comfort zone. And the more we share, the more we will help our mitras to navigate their own experiences.

Remember to begin and end your mitra meetings with the mantra "Protect us together. Nourish us together. May our knowledge and strength ever increase. May we never misunderstand one another. Om peace, peace, peace. *Om saha navavatu…*"

Key Terms from Week Two

Yogini: Female yogi.

Avidya: Delusion, confusion.

Ragah: Attachment.

Dvesha: Aversion, anger.

Asmita: Pride, ego, isolation, loneliness.

Abhinivesha: Fear.

Irshya: Jealousy.

Sharm: Shame.

Dukkha: Depression, sorrow.

Chintashoonyam: Anxiety.

SUBTLE BODY, PHYSICAL BODY

Understand How Thoughts and Emotions
Affect Your Health and Reality

The question is not whether the mind can regulate physiology,
but whether we can regulate the mind.

EKNATH EASWARAN

Yoga is rooted in a profound understanding of the mind-body connection. The mind — which consists of our thoughts and emotions — determines our health, vitality, and the possibility of realizing our svadharma (purpose and potential).

The Upanishads and Bhagavad Gita describe the lower mind as the part of the mind that is conditioned, automatic, and reactive. When someone yells at us and we yell right back, we are functioning from the lower mind. The higher mind is discerning. From here, we consciously choose our thoughts, words, and actions. When operating from the higher mind, if someone yells at us, we pause, breathe, and do our best to respond in a way that helps the situation instead of causing further harm.

As I mentioned in the introduction, in yoga principles, the body consists of five layers or sheaths, which are referred to as the physical, energetic, mental, conscious, and bliss bodies. These five layers are called *koshas* in Sanskrit and are described in the Taittiriya Upanishad, which dates back to the fifth or sixth century BCE.

The outermost layer is the *physical body*, or *annamaya kosha*. This is the layer we are familiar with and that we see each time we look in the mirror.

Below this is the *energetic body*, or *pranamaya kosha*. We can't see the energetic body, but we can feel it. For example, we can't see *prana* — the vital energy inside the breath — but we can feel the healing effects of breathing slowly and deeply versus in a shallow and fast manner. This difference is well researched and accepted within the medical field. In addition to prana, this layer also includes energy channels (*nadis*), pranic winds (*vayus*), and energy centers (*chakras*), all of which are discussed later in this chapter.

The third layer of the body is the lower mind or *mental body*, the *manomaya kosha*, mentioned above, which operates on autopilot. It encompasses mental patterns that influence how we perceive and react to external stimuli. By recognizing and addressing these patterns within the mental layer, we gain insight into our conditioned patterns, setting the stage for deeper work.

The fourth layer is the discerning, higher mind or *wisdom body*, the *vijnanamaya kosha*. This kosha involves our ability to reason and make decisions based on a deeper understanding of life's truths. It is here that we address and transform conditioned patterns, integrating wisdom and applying it in meaningful ways. The mind training at the heart of yoga takes place in this fourth layer.

Depending on our habitual responses, we may experience what lies in the fifth layer: bliss, or *anandamaya kosha*. This deepest layer is a space of ever-present peace and possibility. As we connect with and rest in this layer, dormant creative and healing energies awaken and surface, revealing our deepest truths and creative potential.

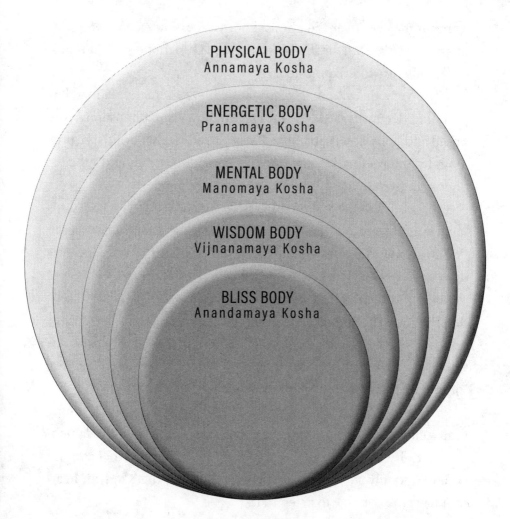

FIGURE 4: The koshas.

Of the five layers of the body described above, only the first is physical; the remaining four are aspects of the subtle body, which in Sanskrit is called *sukshma sarira*. Thoughts and emotions are the food of the subtle body and influence its many elements. Yoga philosophy, as well as other Eastern traditions such as Taoism, acknowledges that by understanding and mastering the subtle body, we gain mastery over the physical body. In essence, *the subtle body determines the state of the physical body*. Our thoughts, emotions, and health are interconnected.

The very definition of *body* in Vedic texts reveals an understanding deeply embedded and explored in Vedic philosophy: The mind and body are inseparable. Physical and mental health are profoundly intertwined. Contemporary clinical research and practice increasingly validate this holistic understanding.

In 2006, while working alongside Dr. Mitchell Gaynor, a pioneer in integrative oncology, I witnessed firsthand how stress, harmful environments, and unprocessed emotions can significantly influence health. Dr. Gaynor emphasized how our thoughts and emotions directly affect our gene expression and overall vitality, highlighting the importance of aligning our inner truth with our external choices. He made groundbreaking strides in using chemotherapy and radiation with integrative therapies such as mantra, pranayama, meditation, gentle asana, and nutrition.*

In a 2015 lecture, Dr. Gaynor stated: "Everything you're thinking and feeling is affecting your gene expression — the most fundamental part of what keeps you healthy, vibrant, alive. So I'd encourage you to not only get more in touch with the truth that's in your heart but have the courage to listen to it."

From a subtle body perspective, the purpose of yoga is to overcome the grip of kleshas, loosen granthis (knots in the subtle body), and liberate prana. Then, prana can move up the central channel, called *sushumna nadi* — the "gracious" or "harmonious"

---

* Dr. Gaynor is the author of several books, including *The Healing Power of Sound* (1999), *Dr. Gaynor's Cancer Prevention Program* (1999), *Healing Essence* (2000), *Nurture Nature, Nurture Health* (2005), and *The Gene Therapy Plan* (2015).

channel — without obstruction. The central channel lies in front of the spine.

When all the granthis are loosened and prana flows freely up the central channel, we can literally hear our song — our knowing, creativity, purpose, and deepest insights. Wisdom comes to us from the inside out. We experience energy and clarity that help us align our thoughts, words, and actions with our most profound truths.

There is an axiom from ancient India: We can be dealt a terrible hand of cards and still play a great game, or we can be dealt an amazing set of cards and play horribly. Our destiny is determined by the choices we make.

To experience the deep satisfaction of knowing and honoring who we truly are, we must work through our kleshas so they don't drain our energy and block our potential. In today's fast-paced world, we often seek quick fixes that rarely provide lasting solutions and can sometimes worsen emotional, mental, and physical issues. Yoga teaches us that true transformation takes time. Its benefits unfold gradually, encouraging us to refine our thoughts, work with our emotions, and take responsibility for how we respond to life's challenges. This journey calls for us to cultivate the qualities of a spiritual warrior, which include:

- A fierce determination
- An indomitable will
- Honesty
- Courage
- Daring
- Discipline
- Focus
- Patience
- Perseverance

A Deeper Exploration of the Subtle Body

Focused on the senses and body, we come to think we are a purely physical entity that can be satisfied through physical means. It is a colossal fallacy that has cost the modern world its health and peace.

EKNATH EASWARAN

We will now explore the subtle body in greater depth and how our thoughts and emotions fuel it. While emotions and thoughts affect the whole body, certain ones significantly influence specific areas. Early yogis had a refined understanding of how particular emotions and thought patterns influence specific aspects of the energetic body, which in turn impact the physical body in distinct ways. This insight can profoundly inform our yoga practices, guiding us to develop emotional and mental resilience alongside physical vitality.

Prana: Vital Force

Beneath the physical body is the energetic or "pranic" body, which, as the name suggests, is comprised of prana. *Prana* is often translated as "breath," but it refers to the vital energy, life force, or spirit within the breath.

Prana is also defined as "the unseen intelligence of the universe" or "the hidden wisdom of the body." The moment my daughter, Mila, was born, she was placed on my belly. On her own, she inched toward my breast and began to nurse. This helped my uterus contract, decrease its bleeding, and return to its normal size. No one whispered into Mila's ear and told her where, how, and when to nurse. Prana — this unseen wisdom — moved through her, as it does in each of us and in all of life.

Prana moves through us every day — as we digest our food, with each respiration, and as the foundation of our alive and self-regulating body. Prana moves through the world, making flowers bloom, rivers flow, and seeds sprout. It's the vital force that exists in all of creation. Through yoga practices, we remove the blocks we carry within so that prana can move through us without obstruction.

In many languages, the word for *breath* and *spirit* is the same, reflecting their fundamental connection. In Latin, "spirit" and "breath" are both rendered as *spiritus*, and in Hebrew, they're called *ruach*. In Portuguese, the word for taking a breath translates as "inspiration," or "spirit in." *Prana* is similar in meaning to the Chinese word *chi* or *qi*, the Japanese term *ki*, and the ancient Egyptian word *ka*.

Central to all yoga practices is the movement and management of prana. By learning to enhance and direct its flow, we strengthen and open the mind and body and develop higher states of awareness.

Vayus: Winds

There are five main movements of prana. They are called *vayus* or "winds." Awareness of these vayus helps us gain optimal benefits from our yoga practices. Vedic texts, including the Yoga Upanishads and Ayurvedic texts, describe how thoughts and emotions influence the movement and balance of these subtle winds, impacting overall health and vitality.

Below is a breakdown of the five winds and the kleshas that most affect them (see figure 5).

- *Prana vayu*, located in the region of the heart and lungs, governs respiration and perception, and is disturbed by anger, resentment, and sorrow.
- *Apana vayu*, a downward-moving wind located in the lower abdomen, influences reproductive organs and governs elimination — including excretion, urination, and menstruation. It is disturbed by fear and isolation.
- *Samana vayu* moves through the digestive organs, aids

digestion and assimilation, and is disturbed by jealousy, confusion, and lack of willpower.

- *Udana vayu*, an upward-moving wind located at the throat, governs growth, speech, and higher states of awareness. It affects the nervous system and is disturbed by attachment, addiction, and shame.
- *Vyana vayu* pervades the entire system. It governs circulation and coordinates all bodily functions, including the lymph and muscular systems. It is disturbed by anxiety and delusion.

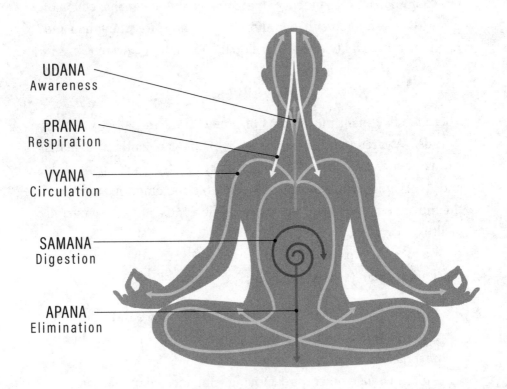

UDANA
Awareness

PRANA
Respiration

VYANA
Circulation

SAMANA
Digestion

APANA
Elimination

FIGURE 5: The five vayus.

When I was going through a divorce, I began to notice that every time I saw a happy couple, especially with a small child close to my daughter's age, I would experience deep pangs of jealousy. Once, I spent an entire night with my mind overcome with jealousy. With my mind endlessly ruminating, I barely slept that night.

The following morning, I felt utterly sick to my stomach. I remembered the teachings about how jealousy affects samana vayu, the pranic winds that move through the digestive organs. I took myself through a yoga practice with poses, breathing exercises, meditations, and visualizations that specifically affect samana vayu. Within an hour, the ill feeling in my stomach was gone. I was amazed. I would never have known how effective the practices are if I hadn't gone through such personal struggles myself.

It's not that I never had moments of jealousy again. I did, and I repeated those practices many times. But from that day onward, I primed my mind to rejoice for happy couples instead of feeling envious of them. The results were incredible. Instead of jealousy tearing me apart inside, creating havoc among my pranic winds, feeling happy for other people's happiness loosened the granthis in my belly and uplifted my spirit. Each time I saw a joyful couple or family, I would not only rejoice for them, I silently thanked them for showing me what was possible. Over many months of rejoicing for and thanking happy couples and families, I started to regain a sense of self-worth. I began to change my thoughts: *If it's possible for them, one day it can be my reality too.* Instead of wallowing in self-pity, my mind opened to acceptance and possibility.

Chakras: Energy Centers

There are seven main chakras, or energy centers (see figure 6), and they are especially susceptible to granthis, or blocks. Unlocking these areas can be profoundly transformative, leading to a freer flow of prana and greater spiritual and psychological well-being. The flow of prana through the chakras is influenced by specific thoughts and emotions.

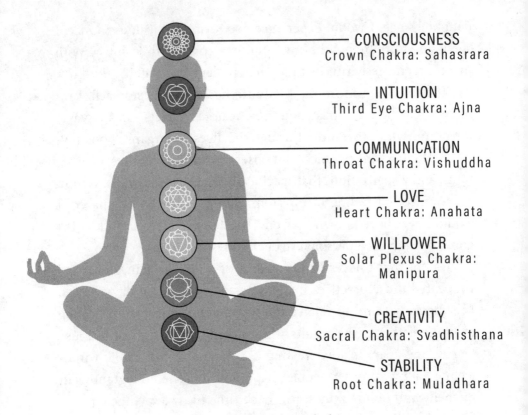

CONSCIOUSNESS
Crown Chakra: Sahasrara

INTUITION
Third Eye Chakra: Ajna

COMMUNICATION
Throat Chakra: Vishuddha

LOVE
Heart Chakra: Anahata

WILLPOWER
Solar Plexus Chakra:
Manipura

CREATIVITY
Sacral Chakra: Svadhisthana

STABILITY
Root Chakra: Muladhara

FIGURE 6: The seven chakras.

1. **Root chakra (*muladhara*)**, located at the base of the spine, governs survival, safety, and stability. A lack of discipline and the kleshas of fear and delusion can block this chakra.

2. **Sacral chakra (*svadhisthana*)**, located below the belly button, is associated with creativity, sexuality, and pleasure. Poor boundaries and the kleshas of shame and isolation often lead to blocks in this chakra.

3. **Solar plexus chakra (*manipura*)**, located above the navel, is responsible for willpower and confidence. Weak will, low self-esteem, and the kleshas of jealousy and anxiety can block this chakra.

4. **Heart chakra (*anahata*)**, located in the chest, governs

relationships, love, self-acceptance, and compassion. A lack of empathy and the kleshas of anger and sorrow can block this energy center.

5. **Throat chakra (*vishuddha*)**, located at the throat, governs communication and expression. Blocks can be caused by lies, an inability to listen, fear of being honest, and primarily the kleshas of attachment and shame.

6. **Third eye chakra (*ajna*)**, associated with the pineal gland and located about an inch above the midpoint between the eyebrows, is responsible for intuition, imagination, and deeper states of awareness. It can be blocked by denial, difficulty concentrating, and the klesha of delusion.

7. **Crown chakra (*sahasrara*)**, located at the top of the head, governs wisdom and spiritual connection. Limited beliefs, materialism, and the kleshas of ego and attachment can block this chakra.

Science on the Mind-Body Connection

Our positive and negative beliefs not only impact our health but also every aspect of our life.

DR. BRUCE LIPTON, *The Biology of Belief*

Scientific research increasingly supports what ancient yogic wisdom has long taught: Our mental and emotional states deeply influence our physical health. Studies in neuroscience, psychology, and epigenetics show that our thoughts, emotions, and beliefs profoundly influence our health, behavior, and life experiences. Both science and spiritual traditions affirm that changing our thoughts reshapes our perceptions, reality, and the way we respond to the world. For instance, neuroscientists have shown how the amygdala — the main area of the brain associated with anger, anxiety, and fear — becomes smaller in meditators. Participants of such studies didn't change anything in their environment. They changed themselves — the way they respond to their environment.

Additional studies show that emotions such as anger, jealousy, shame, anxiety, fear, and depression can lead to adverse health outcomes, including weakened immune functioning, cardiovascular issues, and increased risk of chronic conditions like heart disease and dementia. For example, shame is linked to negative changes in the immune and cardiovascular systems. Loneliness significantly heightens the risk of heart disease, stroke, and dementia. Anger and anxiety disorders are associated with higher risk of cardiovascular diseases.

Conversely, emotions tied to love, hope, connection, worthiness, joy, and peace have been shown to enhance physical health. Compassion is connected to improved mood and decreased blood pressure, stress, and loneliness. Inner peace is associated with a slower heart rate, lower cholesterol, slower aging, reduced anxiety, and healthier immune functioning. Whereas low self-worth can contribute to poor concentration, fatigue, irritability, insomnia, and depression, greater self-worth is linked to improved well-being and life satisfaction. Optimism is associated with an 11 to 15 percent longer lifespan.

A study on the placebo effect published in the *Journal of Neuroscience* revealed how a person's thoughts and beliefs about the effectiveness of a treatment can trigger the release of endorphins and other neurotransmitters, resulting in significant pain reduction. Numerous scientific studies provide evidence suggesting that beliefs and emotions such as positive expectations and optimism can lead to better health outcomes, such as lower levels of inflammation, healthier lipid profiles, and better immune function and cardiovascular health.

These scientific insights align with yogic teachings that thoughts and emotions shape our health. Tailored sequences of movement, breathing techniques, visualization, contemplation, and mantra can deepen our understanding of the subtle body and help us navigate through specific kleshas. This approach lies at the heart of the Yogi's Way.

The Power of Visualization

When we believe we can heal ourselves, it makes a difference. When we start to link our health with our thoughts, we can visualize what we want to experience and send the body messages to heal. There is specific research demonstrating how visualization can improve various aspects of physical well-being, including pain management, stress reduction, immune function, cardiovascular health, and rehabilitation. Numerous studies have also shown that the power of visualization can lead to dramatic improvements in sports performance, skill acquisition, and goal achievement. For example, visualization is a way for athletes to mentally rehearse movements and strategies, leading to enhanced skill development, confidence, and focus. In addition, visualizing goals has been shown to increase motivation and persistence. Studies have found that individuals who vividly imagine themselves succeeding in their goals — whether related to athletics, health, or healing — are more likely to take action and overcome obstacles to achieve their desired outcomes.

It takes practice and repetition for visualization to have such powerful impacts. *Neuroplasticity* refers to the brain's ability to change and adapt. Studies in neuroplasticity reveal that altering our behavior requires repetition. When we do something new, we create new neural pathways in the brain. We have to do the same thing again and again for those neural pathways to become established. As they are, new habits are created, and old ones fall away. The shape of our brain changes, as do our perceptions and personal reality. It is no wonder that yogis emphasize a daily and consistent practice filled with repetition. This is how lasting change occurs.

Research in neuroplasticity reveals that if we change a habitual thought pattern, such as *I'm not good enough* to *My gifts are important*, we forge new neural connections in the brain that reinforce those positive thought patterns. As it is often summarized, "Neurons that wire together fire together."

Considering the extensive findings that correlate mental states with health, we can appreciate the immense value of yoga practices, which are rooted in a philosophy of positive thinking. Visualization is one of the twelve pillars of the Yogi's Way listed on pages 12–13. To be effective, each of these twelve pillars requires practice and repetition. Through daily practice, we cultivate new and empowering thought patterns while releasing harmful ones that we may have carried for decades or even generations. By the end of this twelve-week program, we will have explored each of the twelve pillars in depth and cultivated a reliable daily practice.

I fear not the man who has practiced 10,000 kicks once,
but I fear the man who has practiced one kick 10,000 times.

BRUCE LEE

Through visualization and yoga's other contemplative practices, we become acutely aware of our thought patterns and perceptions. How can we change our thoughts to live our best life? This is a timeless inquiry that we will continue to explore throughout this book.

Yoga from the Inside Out and the Outside In

Just as one's state of mind affects the body, the state of the body also affects the mind. It's vital for the mind to think constructive, nurturing, positive thoughts to make the body healthier. It's also important for the body to exercise regularly, receive proper nutrition, and have adequate time for rest and relaxation. Many of us lead sedentary lives in today's digital world, so it is especially important that we move our bodies every day. For optimal health, yogis practice from the inside out (working with thoughts to affect physical reality) *and* from the outside in (working with the physical body and the breath to open pathways to the innermost Self). With this in mind, in the remaining sections of this book, we will engage in practices to replace destructive thoughts with beneficial ones, as well as movement practices to cultivate a strong and resilient body.

Prepare for Your Practices

The time you set aside for your breath, movement, and journaling practices is a special period for you to water the seeds of possibility within yourself. To prepare, take a warm shower or bath. Wear fresh, loose clothes. Make sure your practice space is clean. Light a candle. Open a window. Let there be natural light and fresh air. Make sure the room isn't too cold, breezy, or hot. Write your motivation from Week One on a piece of paper and place it where you can see it in your practice space. Feel free to refine or rewrite it, if you like. After you review your motivation, ask for blessings like you did in Week One (page 29), and begin your practices.

Week Three Practices

1. Subtle Body Awareness

Review the vayus section on pages 55–56 and in table 1 below. Then, draw a simple picture of yourself with the five main vayus. Considering how each vayu is affected by a certain set of emotions, ask yourself which vayus within you may be the most blocked. Write down the two vayus that you feel you most need to work with.

Table 1. The Vayus and Their Functions

Vayu	Parts of the Body	Functions	Movement	Kleshas
Prana	Chest, heart, lungs, head, respiratory system	Respiration, reception (air, food, impressions, ideas), energizing force	Inward moving in region of lungs and heart	Anger, resentment, sorrow
Apana	Lower abdomen, reproductive organs, excretory system	Elimination, supports immune system	Downward and outward	Isolation, fear
Samana	Navel, digestive system	Digestion; assimilation of physical, mental, and emotional experiences; brings balance and transformation	Expansive, with the potential to awaken the central channel	Jealousy, confusion
Udana	Throat, thyroid and parathyroid glands, nervous system	Speech, expression, metabolism, higher consciousness	Upward, from heart and throat to brain	Attachment, addiction, shame
Vyana	Entire body, particularly the limbs and skin; coordinates all bodily functions, especially circulatory, lymph, muscular, and nervous systems	Helps balance and nourish the other four vayus to bring healing energy throughout the mind and body	Entire system	Anxiety, isolation, delusion

Next, review the chakras section on pages 58–59 and in table 2 below. Then, draw another simple figure of yourself. Place seven circles where the seven main chakras are located. After reviewing which emotions affect each chakra, identify two chakras that you feel may be the most obstructed.

Table 2. The Chakras and Their Functions

Chakra	Location	Functions	Kleshas
Root (muladhara)	Base of spine	Survival: to be here, to have, to be grounded	Fear, delusion
Sacral (svadhisthana)	Below the navel	Emotions, sexuality: to feel, to want	Shame, isolation
Solar plexus (manipura)	Navel	Willpower, confidence: to act, to have purpose	Jealousy, anxiety
Heart (anahata)	Heart	Relationships: to love, to be loved	Anger, sorrow
Throat (vishuddha)	Throat	Communication: to speak, to be heard	Attachment, shame
Third eye (ajna)	Between the eyebrows; pineal gland	Intuition: to see, to imagine, to intuit	Delusion
Crown (sahasrara)	Top of head	Wisdom: to know, to connect to ultimate truth directly	Ego, attachment

2. Ujjayi Pranayama: Victorious Breath

When the breath wanders, the mind is unsteady.
When the breath is steady, so is the mind.

HATHA YOGA PRADIPIKA

Let's set the foundation for your movement practice: the breath, specifically a breath called *ujjayi pranayama*. Translated as "victorious breath" and sometimes also referred to as "ocean breath" because of its sound, ujjayi is the breath pattern typically used while practicing any asana.

Ujjayi is a type of diaphragmatic breath. The diaphragm controls the length and speed of the breath and is strengthened through breathing. The inhales and exhales in ujjayi are through the nose, are of equal duration, and cause no distress to the practitioner. Following James Nestor's research in *Breath: The New Science of a Lost Art*, we will aim for a six-second inhale and a six-second exhale. Especially if you are a beginner, feel free to begin this practice with a two-, three-, four-, or five-second inhale and exhale. With practice, the length of the breath will increase. Take your time to become familiar with ujjayi breath before incorporating it into the movement practice. While breathing in and out through the nose, narrow the throat passage by slightly contracting it. This creates an ocean sound at the back of the throat while you are breathing.

Here's how to do it:

1. Draw the air in through the nose. The air travels to the back of the throat, enters the lungs, expands and lifts the rib cage, and lengthens the intercostal muscles. Intercostal muscles are groups of muscles between the ribs that help form and move the chest wall.

2. As you exhale through the nose, notice the abdomen naturally move in. Slightly contract the muscles of the lower abdomen to assist the air to fully exit the lungs before your next inhale. Maintain a slight contraction of the muscles in the lower abdomen as you inhale.

3. Repeat until you have a smooth, continuous flow of breath.

Practice Tips

•   If the breath is restricted, you are contracting the abdomen too much. Allow the contraction to be subtle.

•   Notice where your breath naturally stops after the exhalation, then exhale a little more than you think you can. Make sure the lungs are completely empty of air before taking the next inhale.

•   Once you incorporate movement, as you move in and out of the poses, maintain a long, deep, and even inhale and exhale. Such rhythmic breathing will support your movement practice to be meditative, grounding, and relaxing.

3. Sun Salutations: A Twelve-Step Movement Practice

The classic twelve-step Surya Namaskara, or Sun Salutation, sequence offers a full-body movement practice. Take your time to become familiar with these twelve poses.

Set aside twenty minutes for this sequence, allowing fifteen minutes for movement and five minutes for rest. Practice at least three rounds of Sun Salutations six times a week. Recall the power of repetition to create new neural pathways and bring lasting change in your mind, body, and life. In the coming weeks, we will also add affirmations in the form of mantras to this movement practice.

Choose a time for your movement practice. The ideal times to practice Surya Namaskara are in the early morning, as the sun rises, or in the evening, as the sun sets. Practicing at the same time every day will yield the best results, but adjust the time if needed.

On a physical level, practicing Sun Salutations lubricates the joints and stretches, tones, massages, and stimulates the major muscle groups and vital organs, helping to revitalize the body and eliminate disease. When practiced with mantra and subtle body awareness, they also have the depth of a spiritual practice that connects us to the possibilities and powers that lie within. To experience the effectiveness of this ancient practice, doing it daily is important. The twelve poses in the sequence are practiced in a steady rhythm that reflects the rhythms of the universe, such as the twenty-four hours of the day, the twelve months of the year, and the biorhythms of our body. As we practice, we generate prana, the vital energy that activates and purifies the body and mind.

As when starting any new exercise program, consult your physician before you begin, especially if you have high blood pressure, coronary artery disease, hernias, intestinal tuberculosis, spinal problems, or sciatica or have had a stroke. During a light menstrual flow, it is OK to practice Surya Namaskara. If your cycle is heavy or painful, it may be best to take a break and let the body rest. Unless there are complications, it is generally safe to practice Surya Namaskara during the first trimester of pregnancy and following childbirth.

The foundation of each asana, or pose, is a relaxed state. As you read the instructions below, take the time to learn each asana by itself. Keep your shoulders, jaw, and muscles of the face relaxed while in each pose. Avoid strain and stay connected to your breath. Your breath is your primary focus, while the pose is secondary. Use your breath to initiate each movement. Allow your breathing to sustain the movement.

While learning the twelve postures, feel free to let yourself remain in each pose for three to five breaths. For example, you can stand in Mountain, the first pose, for several breaths and then inhale the arms up into pose 2, Raised Arms Pose. Keep breathing with the arms stretched up and back as you lift your heart. Then, exhale into pose 3, Forward Bend, and feel free to remain in this position for a few breaths before inhaling into pose 4, Low Lunge. Do this with each pose.

It is beneficial to practice slowly, especially in the beginning. As you become familiar with the movements, the practice may naturally evolve to one breath per movement. After you have practiced several times and are familiar with the breathing and movement techniques, allow the mind to rest by focusing on the soothing sound of your ujjayi breathing, the ocean breath.

Having practiced Surya Namaskara for several decades, I still have days when I stay for a few breaths in each pose. On such days, I simply feel like moving slowly. On other days, practicing at the pace of one breath per movement feels great. There isn't a right, wrong, better, or worse way. It's just a matter of being with what feels right each day. Both have benefits. For example, moving slowly can build more strength. Moving at the pace of one breath per movement can build more energy if you're feeling lethargic. Be present and honor your needs and intuition in the moment. Once you get to know the sequence, you can practice with eyes closed or open. Make this choice according to what helps you stay most focused.

For video instruction, see TheYogisWay.com/thebook.

SUN SALUTATION PRACTICE

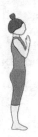

1. Mountain Pose
(Tadasana)

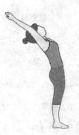

2. Raised Arms Pose
(Hasta Uttanasana)

3. Forward Bend
(Uttanasana)

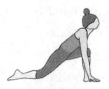

4. Equestrian Pose
or Low Lunge
(Ashwa Sanchalanasana)

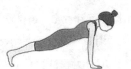

5. Plank Pose
(Phalakasana)

6. Eight Points Salute
(Ashtanga Namaskara)

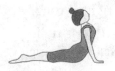

7. Cobra Pose
(Bhujangasana)

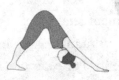

8. Downward-Facing Dog
(Adho Mukha Svanasana)

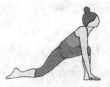

9. Equestrian Pose
or Low Lunge
(Ashwa Sanchalanasana)

10. Forward Bend
(Uttanasana)

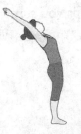

11. Raised Arms Pose
(Hasta Uttanasana)

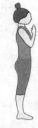

12. Mountain Pose
(Tadasana)

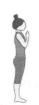

1. **Mountain Pose (Tadasana):** Stand at the front of the yoga mat or practice space, facing the direction of the sun. Place the feet together or hip width apart. Bring your palms together at the heart or allow your arms to rest straight and relaxed by your sides with the palms turned out. Relax the entire body, grounding the feet down toward the center of the earth as you extend the crown of the head toward the sky. Breathe in and out.

2. **Raised Arms Pose (Hasta Uttanasana):** Inhale and raise the arms up and back to lift the heart and arch the back. Keep shoulders relaxed, away from the ears. If the shoulders are tight, allow the arms to be shoulder width apart. Otherwise, keep the palms of the hands together. Gaze up at the thumbs.

3. **Forward Bend (Uttanasana):** Exhale as you bend forward, bringing your hands to your shins, ankles, the floor, or yoga blocks. Soften the knees to ease any tension in the lower back. Relax the shoulders and neck. As you expel the air from the lungs, gently contract the abdomen. Gaze toward the tip of your nose.

4. **Equestrian Pose or Low Lunge (Ashwa Sanchalanasana):** Inhale, bend your knees, place your hands flat on the floor, and step your right foot back into a high lunge. Drop the right knee down to the ground. Gaze forward or up to the sky. Lift the heart and relax the shoulders down. If placing the hands flat is challenging, place your fingertips on the ground, support your hands on blocks, or raise your arms up to the sky.

5. **Plank Pose (Phalakasana):** Exhale and step your left foot back to meet the right. Keep your shoulders over your wrists and your feet hip width apart. Keep the back of the neck straight. Pull the navel upward.

6. **Eight Points Salute (Ashtanga Namaskara):** Hold the breath and lower your knees to the floor. Then bring your chest and chin to the ground, keeping the buttocks elevated.

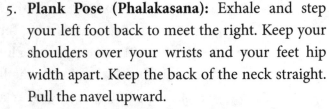

7. **Cobra Pose (Bhujangasana):** Inhale, lower the hips, and extend the legs with your feet together and the toes flat against the floor. Lift the chest forward and up. Pull the shoulders back and gaze forward or up.

8. **Downward-Facing Dog (Adho Mukha Svanasana):** Exhale and lift the hips up while pressing the hands into the earth. Spread the fingers wide. Lengthen the back and gently pull the heels downward. Soften the gaze toward the navel. Relax the shoulders. Soften the knees if the backs of the legs feel tight.

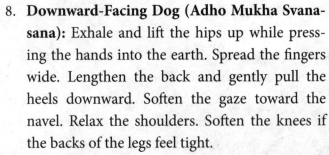

9. **Equestrian Pose or Low Lunge (Ashwa Sanchalanasana):** Inhale and step the right foot forward between the hands. Gaze forward or up if this does not strain the neck.

10. **Forward Bend (Uttanasana):** Exhale and bend forward at the waist. Place the hands on the shins, ankles, earth, or yoga blocks. Bring the head toward the knees. Gaze toward the tip of the nose.

11. **Raised Arms Pose (Hasta Uttanasana):** Inhale, gently raise the arms up and back, and lift the heart. Gaze forward or up.

12. **Mountain Pose (Tadasana):** Exhale as you bring your hands down by your sides or place your palms together at the heart. Relax and breathe.

Practice Tips

- Practice each pose with minimum effort, moving and stretching in the most efficient and enjoyable way while conserving energy.
- If you find the transition from pose 3 to pose 4 difficult, break the sequence down into two sets. First, practice only poses 1, 2, 3, 11, and 12. Then, practice only 4, 5, 6, 7, 8, and 9. Once these two stages are comfortable for you, combine them for the full sequence.
- If moving from pose 7 to pose 8 is too difficult, after pose 7, bring your hands and knees to the floor and then shift to pose 8. Figure 7 illustrates this transition between poses 7 and 8.

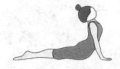
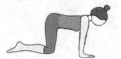
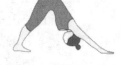

7. Cobra Pose
(Bhujangasana)

8. Downward-Facing Dog
(Adho Mukha Svanasana)

FIGURE 7: Modified transition between poses 7 and 8.

- If the complete series of twelve poses feels too difficult, another way to modify it is by reducing it to a nine-posture sequence. First, move through poses 1 to 4, then poses 8 to 12.
- Always avoid strain, especially if you are elderly or healing from an injury. If you are a beginner, start by becoming comfortable with three rounds of the sequence.

- I recommend not playing music during your Sun Salutation practice. Instead, give yourself the gift of silence, which is increasingly rare in our modern world. Listen inward to the ocean sound of your ujjayi breath. Feel the sensation of your breath as it moves in and out of your body and as it moves you in and out of each pose. Silence is powerful. As you engage in your practices, be completely present with your body, breath, heart, and soul.

Silence is to the soul what water is to the body.

ANONYMOUS

4. Sun Salutations with Chakra Awareness

Once you feel comfortable with ujjayi breath and the twelve poses of Surya Namaskara, begin to add chakra awareness to your Sun Salutation practice. In each pose, focus on the chakra associated with that pose as described on the next page. Drawing attention to the chakras helps develop concentration and activates the chakras, increasing their functioning. Again, feel free to remain in each pose for several breaths.

One approach you could take this week is to practice ujjayi breath with the twelve poses for the first three days. Then, add chakra awareness for the remaining three days of practice.

SUN SALUTATION WITH CHAKRA AWARENESS

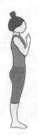

1. Inhale and exhale.
Mountain Pose. *Heart chakra:*
acceptance, compassion,
to love and be loved.

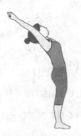

2. Inhale. Raised Arms
Pose. *Throat chakra:*
to speak and be heard.

3. Exhale. Forward
Bend. *Sacral chakra:*
to feel and to want.

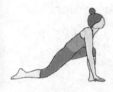

4. Inhale, right foot back.
Low Lunge. *Third eye chakra:*
to see, imagine, intuit.

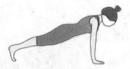

5. Exhale, left foot back.
Plank Pose. *Throat chakra:*
to speak and be heard.

6. Retaining breath, lower knees,
chest, and chin. Eight Points Salute.
Solar plexus chakra: to act with
confidence and will.

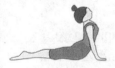

7. Inhale. Cobra Pose.
Sacral chakra:
to feel and to want.

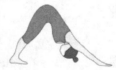

8. Exhale, lift hips.
Downward-Facing Dog. *Throat*
chakra: to speak and be heard.

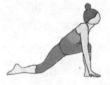

9. Inhale, right foot forward.
Low Lunge. *Third eye chakra:*
to see, imagine, intuit.

10. Exhale, left foot forward.
Forward Bend. *Sacral chakra:*
to feel and to want.

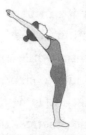

11. Inhale. Raised Arms
Pose. *Throat chakra: to*
speak and be heard.

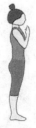

12. Exhale. Mountain Pose.
Heart chakra: acceptance,
compassion, to love and be loved.

5. Rest

Always end your practice with the yoga pose of complete relaxation, Savasana, which translates to "Corpse Pose." Lie on your back with legs and hands extended. The palms face the sky, and the feet fall naturally to the sides. Close your eyes and draw your awareness inward. Relax every part of your body, from your feet to the crown of your head. Allow the mind to rest. Let your breathing be natural. Stay in this pose for five minutes, allowing your heartbeat and breath to return to a restful state. During these five minutes, visualize your chakras opening and prana moving smoothly through them. In ancient texts, each chakra is depicted as a flower. Like flowers, chakras can close or open.

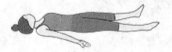

FIGURE 8: Savasana, or Corpse Pose.

Visualization is powerful when we put the work and time into making the changes we envision. Now that you've completed your Sun Salutations while being aware of your breath and chakras, visualize your body opening to your deepest, wisest, most true Self. With the chakras open, also see yourself as receptive to life's blessings.

Savasana invites contemplation of death, acknowledging its inevitability and the fact that it can happen at any moment. This awareness serves as an inspiration to keep practicing so we can uncover and honor our full potential while we inhabit the body.

After Savasana, take a minute to stand under the sun and take in its rays or go for a short walk and let your body, mind, heart, and spirit continue to assimilate the practice. Throughout the world, indigenous cultures have had a tradition of opening their bodies and minds to receive the sun's energy. I invite you to feel connected to this rich history.

6. Journaling

When you are ready, before moving on with all the things you have to do today, spend five or ten minutes writing in your journal. Reflect on your practice. What did it bring up for you, especially after adding chakra awareness to your breathing and movement? How are you feeling now? Try not to think too much about what you are writing. Just let your expression flow.

Week Three Daily Practice Sequence

1. Optimal Breath practice: five minutes at the beginning of the day
2. All-Day Yoga
3. Sun Salutations with chakra awareness: fifteen minutes
4. Savasana: five minutes
5. Journaling: five to ten minutes
6. Klesha Trigger Log: five to ten minutes at the end of the day

Total daily practice time: thirty-five to forty-five minutes

Week Three Mitra Meeting

Review the five layers of the body with your mitras. What are they and what do they signify? How was your experience drawing your body with the vayus and chakras? How did it feel to practice the twelve-step Sun Salutation sequence with and without awareness of the chakras? Do you need to modify the practice in any way? How? What time have you chosen to practice the Sun Salutations? Share the time you chose with your mitras. Remember, your homework is to practice at least three rounds of Sun Salutations six times a week.

Always follow your Sun Salutations with Savasana. Enjoy relaxing the body entirely and envisioning the chakras opening. Have any questions arisen to debate and discuss?

Key Terms from Week Three

Koshas: The five layers that make up the body.

Sukshma sarira: The subtle body, consisting of the four layers beneath the physical body.

Prana: Vital energy, life force, spirit.

Nadi: Energy channel in the body.

Sushumna nadi: The body's central energy channel.

Vayus: The winds or vital energy currents of the body.

Chakras: The energy centers of the body.

Ujjayi pranayama: A breath pattern used while practicing asana; translates as "victorious breath."

Surya Namaskara: Sun Salutation

CONSCIOUSNESS

Rest, Recover, Strengthen

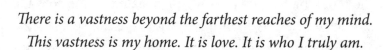

There is a vastness beyond the farthest reaches of my mind.
This vastness is my home. It is love. It is who I truly am.

Sri Nisargadatta Maharaj

In Week One, we identified our mitras and invited them on a journey with us to work through our kleshas and connect with our svadharma (purpose and potential). In Week Two, we defined the major kleshas and acknowledged the ones that may affect us the most. In Week Three, we explored how thoughts and emotions, including kleshas, affect the subtle body, which in turn affects the physical body. We gained insight into why working through kleshas is central to yoga and to our health, healing, and the possibility of realizing our full potential.

This week, we will explore the lens through which we confront our kleshas.

In connection with moving through difficult emotions, you've probably heard the phrases "Feel what you feel" or "Feel it to heal it." It's true that we must experience our emotions — from the pleasant to the painful — wholeheartedly in order to heal. Otherwise, suppressed emotions become larger and heavier, causing damage to our mental and physical health.

Vedic philosophy adds a subtle yet profound element to the practice of being present with our emotions. We meet our present-moment thoughts and emotions from the seat of consciousness — a quiet, spacious, nonjudgmental presence. In this chapter, we will explore the meaning and significance of consciousness, as well as the yogic journey to move from the tumultuous mind and the grip of kleshas to that spacious abode.

Within yoga wisdom traditions, consciousness is unequivocally the most challenging teaching to explain. Yet the goal and the meaning of yoga are to be in union with consciousness. Although no words capture this experience, having an intellectual understanding of it prepares us to experience it directly.

Before diving into the subject of consciousness, I'll first explain an essential lesson in yoga traditions about how to receive a spiritual teaching. The ancient yogis were adamant that we mustn't blindly believe anything a spiritual teacher tells us. "Only believe what you experience" is a principal message of the Upanishads.

To prime ourselves for direct experiences, yogis in the Vedic tradition prescribe a three-step process for receiving a spiritual teaching. First is *shravan*, which means "listening." Yogis are aware of the tendency for the mind to get distracted with self-talk and wandering thoughts, so students are asked to do their best to set aside nonrelevant thoughts and keep the mind focused. While giving your full attention, let the teachings penetrate your heart and mind.

The second step is *manan*, which means "reflection" or "contemplation." After listening to a teaching, allow yourself time to assimilate it. You can ask yourself: How does this teaching resonate with me?

The third step is *nididhyasana*, which means "meditation." Here, we engage in meditative practices to experience truth directly, within our own being. With practice, concepts turn into realizations. For example, a concept that you read or heard, such as "You are pure potential," becomes a direct experience when granthis (knots) open, allowing you to feel that truth within yourself, in every fiber of your being. When a teaching is embodied, it transforms into a living truth, carrying a power that resonates through daily life.

Keeping these three steps in mind, let's begin this week's teaching on consciousness and what it signifies in the Vedic tradition.

1. **Shravan:** listening
2. **Manan:** reflection
3. **Nididhyasana:** meditation for direct experience

Yoga means "to yoke" or "to unite." It connects us to an unchanging reality. *Wait*, you might be thinking, *I thought that everything is changing — that change is the only constant.* Yes, this is true...and there is a deeper reality. Underlying all the ups and downs we inevitably experience in life, there exists a changeless reality that is quiet and infinitely spacious. Buddhists call this unchanging dimension *shunyata*, which means "emptiness." Hindus call it *purna*, which means "fullness." Quantum physicists call it "a field of pure potentiality." Mystics and meditators throughout the world experience this space as love. The Taoists captured this truth with the statement: "The Tao that can be named is not the real Tao."* This deepest reality of consciousness is impossible to describe in words. Naming it or trying to describe it limits its true essence. This is the very reason Vedic texts emphasize direct experience.

The purpose of spiritual practice — and, some would say, the purpose of life itself — is to experience this ultimate truth directly. This isn't meant to be a miraculous, momentary achievement. With practice, we learn to connect with the silent and vast field of consciousness and rest our minds here. As we do, our energy is restored,

---

*   Opening lines of the Tao Te Ching, an ancient Chinese text attributed to the sage Lao Tzu. It reflects the idea that the underlying reality transcends human language and is beyond conceptualization or description.

and our mind and body strengthen. It is from these quiet depths that dormant and blocked creative energies awaken, and we connect with our deepest wisdom. Eventually, we are able to anchor ourselves in consciousness while we engage with the world.

To be in the state of yoga — in union with consciousness — is referred to as *sat-chit-ananda*: the bliss of knowing that the essence of who you are is eternal, infinite, unchanging, and of boundless possibility.* Knowing this dimension is what the Bible may be referring to when it talks about "the peace that passeth all understanding" (Philippians 4:7).

Sri Sri Ravi Shankar compares consciousness to sunlight. Whether sunlight shines on mud or on clear water, the light itself doesn't change. It is unaffected, undisturbed, undefended, and undamageable. From the seat of consciousness, whether we experience pain or pleasure, kleshas or bliss, we remain connected to our innermost being, an unchanging source of love and infinite possibility. Whether we fall on our face a hundred times or sail smoothly through our life challenges, whether we experience praise, criticism, profit, loss, joy, or heartbreak, the love and pure potential at the essence of our being remain. In the state of yoga — yoked with this dimension — it becomes much easier to get up again and again when life gets challenging. Radical resilience comes with being in union with consciousness. The combination of vital energy and love that consciousness exudes is our most potent healer, our greatest champion, our source of energy — and it is right here, at the center of our being.

Ancient Sanskrit texts compare the mind to the sea. The surface is turbulent and chaotic, with constant change and movement. The depths, however, carry a profound stillness, silence, and vastness.

---

*   In the translation of *yoga* as "union with the true Self," the "true Self" does not refer to our individual personalities or gifts. The true Self is the consciousness that exists as the essence of all beings.

This is the possibility of a mind that experiences consciousness. It is expansive and limitless. Our fleeting and repetitive thoughts cease to have a strong hold on us when we are connected to something profound and compelling. We experience moments of insight and revelation from these quiet depths. Furthermore, when anchored in the vastness of consciousness, we can find space to breathe, pause, and intentionally respond to life instead of automatically reacting to it. Here, we connect with our true, peaceful, wise, creative Self and can explore our full human potential.

Becoming a witness to all that is happening in our mind is a stepping stone to experiencing consciousness directly. This is the step we will take this week.

First, let's establish a clear understanding of the difference between the mind's tendencies and the nature of consciousness. Remember, listening and understanding come first. Then, meditative practices help us turn concepts into direct realizations.

Mind versus Consciousness

The mind constantly changes. It fluctuates between the past and future. It judges moments as "good," "bad," "right," "wrong," "better," or "worse." It is constantly on guard, resisting discomfort and chasing pleasure. The mind is often cluttered and restless, filled with repetitive thoughts that drain our energy.

By contrast, consciousness is unchanging. It is always present. Consciousness is quiet in the sense that it doesn't judge or label moments as good, bad, et cetera. A moment simply is what it is. Consciousness is spacious in the sense that there is room for all experience — fear, anger, sorrow, jealousy, profit, loss, victory, defeat, shame, joy. Consciousness is still in the sense that it doesn't push away pain or grasp at pleasure. It allows each emotion, thought, sensation, and experience that arises to be as it is and to come and to go, without fighting, pulling, pushing, or grasping at it. Whatever comes or goes, consciousness is unaffected, remains undisturbed, and cannot be tainted. In these ways, consciousness is infinitely spacious, quiet, and still, like the vastness found at the depths of the sea.

On this path of the Yogi's Way, we engage kleshas from the seat of consciousness — a spacious, welcoming, nonjudgmental presence. When pain arises, there is no resistance. We let it be felt. Resistance is the mind's way of protecting itself from the discomfort of facing the wounds and traumas that kleshas are often born from. When we are grounded in love and spaciousness, we can give kleshas the attention and understanding they need. Any thought or emotion that is met with complete acceptance changes. Its hold on us diminishes. This is the power of nonjudgmental presence.

From the seat of consciousness, we allow ourselves to experience our wholeness — the pleasant and the painful, the kleshas and the joys. After all, the word *healing* comes from the word *whole*.

When small children cry, if we yell at them to stop, they cry louder. If we listen to them and give them space to cry while offering tenderness and affection, their bodies relax in our arms. Their entire being changes. We can see the shift in their faces and body language. This is how we meet our kleshas. This is how the pain begins to transform. Instead of it holding us down, we begin to heal and grow.

The wholehearted acceptance of pain releases
the springs of happiness.

Sri Nisargadatta Maharaj

Be a gracious host even to the most unruly guests.

Tibetan proverb

Many of us were raised without permission to feel the full range of human emotion. For example, women have been shamed for feeling anger and being assertive. Men are not always accepted for feeling vulnerable or afraid. Consciousness opens us to experiencing all our emotions, so we can channel the energy and teachings behind these emotions in healthy ways. For example, anger can show us what is important to us and give us the energy to act and mobilize people if our rights are being violated. Anger itself is not bad. No emotion is good or bad in and of itself. The seat of consciousness that transcends the labels of good, bad, right, and wrong applies to what naturally arises in our emotional field. It does not apply to how we act on these emotions. Anger can lead to horrific outcomes, such as violence and war. On this path, we are learning to experience the full range of emotions and channel them in constructive instead of devastating ways that harm ourselves and others.

Witness Meditation

Be the unseen seer that allows all experience to take place.

SRI RAMANA MAHARSHI

You can listen to this meditation at TheYogisWay.com/thebook.

Silence your notifications on your devices and set your timer for six minutes.

To get a feeling for the dimension of consciousness, sit comfortably on a chair or on the ground. Breathe slowly. Relax your body, especially the shoulders, hips, and face. Lengthen the spine and align the shoulders over the hips. Keep the chin parallel to the ground.

With your eyes closed, bring your attention to your third eye, about an inch above the midpoint of your eyebrows. From here, look at the space behind your forehead. Notice it is boundless. It has no beginning or end. There is a quietness here, a stillness. Whatever arises in this space —a pleasant thought, a painful emotion, a wonderful or uncomfortable sensation — the space itself doesn't change. There's a freedom to be had here, a peace. In this space, there is room for all experience — confusion, clarity, doubt, fear, joy, excitement, compassion, anger.

Become a silent witness to whatever thought, emotion, sensation, or experience arises in this space. Whether it is pleasant or painful, let it be. Give yourself permission to relax, breathe, and be in the moment. Try not to resist an uncomfortable emotion or grasp at a pleasant experience. All thoughts, emotions, sensations, and experiences are temporary. Let them come and go. Be the watcher — the light of consciousness that, like sunlight, doesn't change whether it shines on mud or clear water.

Keep your gaze steady and relaxed on the vast space behind your forehead. Witness all that comes and goes from a quiet, still, nonjudgmental, and welcoming presence.

When the six minutes have passed, journal about your experience. If your mind wandered the entire time, that's OK. Whatever happened, be the silent and gracious witness of your experience.

Table 3 summarizes the tendencies of the mind compared to the nature of consciousness.

Table 3. The Mind versus Consciousness

Mind	Consciousness
Changing	Unchanging
Likes/dislikes	Nonjudgmental
Moves to the past and future	Rests in the present
Rejects pain and grasps pleasure	Allows/accepts everything

Mind	Consciousness
Compares	No comparison
Judges	No judgment
Analyzes	No analysis
Reacts	No reaction
Affected	Unaffected
Restless	Undisturbed
Imprisoned	Open

Table 4 illustrates how findings in the field of neuroscience parallel yogic teachings on the mind and consciousness, particularly in their exploration of the left and right hemispheres of the brain.

Table 4. The Left and Right Hemispheres of the Brain

Left Hemisphere of the Brain	Right Hemisphere of the Brain
Lives through memory and anticipation	Stays in present-moment awareness
Endless preoccupation with memories of the past and imaginings of the future	Fresh, in the now
Experience as a representation of the world, a mental image, rather than what is	Meets the moment as it is

Yogis and scientists agree that aspects of the mind that can be harmful are also sometimes useful. For instance, we need the mind to judge, analyze, and react quickly in life-threatening situations. Similarly, both hemispheres of the brain play important roles. In general, the left hemisphere is associated with analytical and logical thinking, language processing, and sequential tasks. The right hemisphere is linked to creativity, intuition, spatial awareness, and holistic thinking. The relationship between the two hemispheres is complementary. In our modern world, the left hemisphere dominates for most of us, leading to significant stress, anxiety, and illness. As we learn to meditate, we come into the present moment and bring balance to the two hemispheres.

From Mental Turmoil to Consciousness: An Experience

One year after separating from my daughter's father, I was still overcome by kleshas, especially anger. My mind would go back to the past, remembering the beauty of when we first met. I was a slave to the past. I noticed the loops playing over and over in my mind — wanting things to be different than they were and imagining how things could have turned out if only.

Even though my partner and I had been struggling, I hadn't wanted to separate. It took at least a year after the separation for me to recognize how much I was forcing and grasping a relationship that simply wasn't working. My mind was attached to the mental image of what a family is supposed to look like: mother, father, and child living together under one roof.

Anger is the response when attachment doesn't get what it wants.

Venerable Robina Courtin

About two years after the separation, I went to India. I stayed for a month in the ashram of the late Sri Ramana Maharshi, one of India's greatest yogis and most influential teachers on consciousness. People from all over the world stay in his ashram to understand and eventually experience the shift from a tumultuous mind to the still and silent space of consciousness.

I spent that month away from my four-year-old daughter. It was heart-wrenching to be away from her for so long, but it had to happen. I was sinking, and Maharshi pulled me up. At his ashram, I practiced being present. I remembered, through his teachings, to trust life rather than fight against it and to be open and receptive to what it brings.

There were two other yoga instructors at the ashram whom I had connected with through mutual friends. Inspired and supported by them, every day I rolled out my yoga mat at 5:00 a.m. and practiced asana with them until 6:15. We practiced in silence, sometimes following one another's sequences and sometimes doing our own thing, but always supported by our shared presence. From 6:30 to 7:30, we went to the terrace of the building where we were all staying and practiced a particular pranayama sequence together in the fresh morning air. I would then return to my room for a shower and have breakfast at 8:30. At 9:00, I would take a five-minute walk to the ashram and spend the rest of the day and evening meditating, walking, reading, praying, singing mantra, and communing with the teachers, students, and spirit of Sri Ramana Maharshi.

Influenced by the collective energy around me — everyone studying consciousness and trying earnestly to apply it to their lives — I learned to let go and let God, to surrender. I allowed myself to stop trying so hard to change the present moment and instead relax and be receptive to it. My mind had been consumed by the doors I saw closing as I lost my partner, family unit, and home. At Maharshi's ashram, I learned to accept the present moment as it is. Pain. Pleasure. Let it come and let it go. No fighting, grasping, pushing, or pulling. Whatever is, is. Allow life to move through you as it does. No judgment. No labels of good or bad, right or wrong, this way or that. Life simply is. It is happening, and all we have to do is allow it. This is pure being, or what Ramana Maharshi called "pure consciousness."

Consciousness accepts everything and rejects nothing.

Consciousness Heals

After about three weeks at the ashram, I was becoming unlocked. One day, I went to the temple after my morning practices and sat down next to a sculpture of Ramana Maharshi. A young Western woman was next to me wailing loudly. I felt myself getting annoyed. *Doesn't she know her loud crying is disturbing? This is a temple, meant to be quiet. People are sitting, meditating, praying.* I let the thoughts come and go and continued to sit.

After a while, I started crying quietly. Pain was arising, the pain of the separation from my husband. I tried to be a good student. I accepted the pain. I welcomed it. I let it move through my body. I felt the pain with all my being. Before I knew it, I was the one sobbing, almost as loudly as the woman near me whom I had judged just a few minutes earlier! She must have been an angel giving me permission to be with my pain, whatever the outcome.

Time ceased to be. I have no idea how long I sat there. I was shaking with tears. My clothes, my face, and the tissues I held in my hand were soaked. Finally, I quieted and stayed seated. I closed my eyes. No medicine, no complicated yogic technique could have been more powerful than simply letting myself be. I allowed life to move through me without resistance. I allowed pain to arise, and I faced it wholeheartedly, with every fiber of my being. Finally, after years of resisting, grasping, fighting, wanting, and longing, it all released. It was as if the chains that were wrapped around my mind literally dissolved. I felt the granthis behind my heart and along my spine loosen and my subtle body open. *I could breathe.*

On the other side of resistance is liberation — freedom from the tyranny in our own minds.

The soul always knows what to do to heal itself.
The challenge is to silence the mind.

CAROLINE MYSS

Healing Is Infectious

The beauty of consciousness is that we not only allow ourselves to be with what is, we allow others the freedom to have their experience too.

It took me months, if not years, to recognize how I wasn't allowing my daughter's father to have his experience — which, like all experience, is valid. He is allowed to feel what he feels, just like I am.

When I was pregnant and he told me he was scared of becoming a father and being my life partner, I resisted. I didn't want to hear what he was saying. Anger and fear clutched at my heart every time he brought up the subject of living separately. My breath became shallow. I couldn't face him. I couldn't accept him. The truth was painful, and I wanted everything to be different. I couldn't embrace how life was unfolding. I couldn't listen to him when he needed to express himself.

I don't judge myself for experiencing this resistance. It is a deep, primal need for pregnant women to be supported, sheltered, and nurtured. In the field of consciousness, there is space for this too. Consciousness is accepting and understanding even of our resistance and the ways our resistance tries to protect us from pain.

Even now, as I recount these memories, some level of hurt remains. I don't know that time completely heals all wounds. I do know that the more the mind experiences the vastness of consciousness, the more we can experience the pain of our traumas as well as the space around them. With practice this space becomes more expansive, and the mind can more easily rest and surrender to the possibilities that each moment holds.

Years after the separation, I realized that as "wrong" as my ex's feelings seemed to me when I was pregnant and then when our child was small, it was his experience to undergo, his feelings to feel — perhaps a result of his own wounds. There is space for this too. Finally, after returning from India, I was able to sit down and hear him. I could breathe and allow him to be and to express himself, without getting defensive and my mind becoming disturbed.

As I listened, I didn't necessarily like what he said. But I was less attached to the part of my mind that likes and dislikes, more connected to a space of acceptance and possibility. I realized that life didn't have to be the way my mind had been so attached to — mother, father, and child living together under the same roof, he and I in a romantic partnership. I still felt some sorrow about this, but at the same time, my mind was open to things being different. To listen to him without reacting and for him to speak without holding back were the most healing things we could have done for our relationship as we navigated a new chapter of coparenting. In that moment, two minds met with vulnerability, love, and understanding. We each released the other, and what has happened since then has simply been better.

Week Four Practices

1. Witness Meditation: Become Present to Yourself

This week, you'll add the Witness Meditation (see page 85) to your weekly practice. To review, the witness is the bridge to consciousness, because the witness carries the same fundamental qualities as consciousness. Here are some descriptions to make this clearer:

- **Mind:** tends to move to the past and future, judge, label, compare, resist discomfort, chase pleasure, and be in constant motion.
- **Witness:** is present, is nonjudgmental, doesn't compare or label, is infinitely spacious (there is room for all thoughts, emotions, sensations, and experiences), doesn't resist discomfort or grasp pleasure, allows each moment to be as it

is. The witness is unchanging, undisturbed, undefended, and indestructible, like sunlight that isn't affected whether it shines on mud or on clear water.

- **Consciousness:** is an underlying, unchanging reality that is a quiet, infinite field of possibility. All phenomena arise, abide, and dissolve in the space of consciousness. Mystics and meditators throughout the world have experienced consciousness as love, the Divine, God, Atman, Source, and healing and liberating light. These words point us to what is ineffable. Becoming a witness to our experiences is a powerful way to turn this concept into realization.

Each day, practice abiding in witnessing presence for six minutes, using the Witness Meditation instructions earlier in this chapter (page 85). Afterward, journal about your experience. How was it to be present, transparent, and lucidly awake to yourself? What was it like for you to *be* the light that is unaffected and unchanging? Even if your mind was moving the entire time, how was it to witness the mind's movements without judgment? To step away and be the watcher of your mind — the unseen seer that allows all experience to take place — what was this like for you?

This week, practice meeting others from witnessing presence. What is your experience?

2. Psychotherapy and Spirituality

Between 2010 and 2012, I had the opportunity to learn various types of psychotherapy with master therapist Lee Joseph. Lee had been practicing psychotherapy for forty years when I met him. He founded a school on Kauai where he taught several modalities, including somatic, Hakomi, and gestalt therapies. Ironically, Lee was also a student of Sri Ramana Maharshi. He had a remarkable ability to combine Vedic teachings of consciousness with the psychotherapy modalities he taught.

One day, early in our training, Lee said, "Everything you feel is valid. It's OK to feel what you feel. There is no emotion that is good or bad." This was powerful because back then I had a history of pushing away uncomfortable and confusing emotions. To hear Lee's simple yet profound words while in the company of twenty open-minded, vulnerable, and brave students moved me to tears. Caught between two very different cultures my entire life — those of the US and of India — I had often felt that I wasn't allowed to feel, be, dress, speak, talk, walk, or even think according to my deepest truths. It seemed like who I was and what I did was shaped by the ideas of others — Indians, Americans, and everyone in between.

The personal, interpersonal, and transpersonal exercises that Lee taught gave me permission to be as I was and to feel what I felt while my fellow students served as witnesses. Each of them gave me their full presence without judgment.

Lee taught us to sit in the seat of consciousness. With every exercise, the first step was establishing ourselves in the open, welcoming, nonjudgmental presence of consciousness. Every day, we became more familiar with the spacious, loving presence of consciousness.

There is a powerful exercise that Lee taught us early in our training, which I invite you to experience with your mitra. Lee called it WAYEN, standing for "What Are You Experiencing Now?" While this practice is best done in person, you can do it online if necessary.

WAYEN: What Are You Experiencing Now?

Sit face-to-face with your mitra. Take a few slow, deep breaths and anchor yourself in the seat of consciousness — an open, welcoming, nonjudgmental presence. While remaining here, meet whatever arises in the moment without resistance. Remember, with your mitra, you are in a safe and sacred space.

Take a few more deep breaths to ground and relax. Then, gaze into your partner's eyes. With a gentle, grounded voice and a slow cadence, ask your mitra: "What are you experiencing now?"

Maintain calm breathing. Hold space for your mitra to relax and take time to respond. Give your partner 100 percent of your attention, not letting your mind get distracted. Regardless of how your partner responds, your role is to be the spacious and welcoming presence of consciousness. Whether your partner cries or laughs, shares something shallow or deep, talks about a klesha or a joy, your job is to listen, exuding the energy that whatever they say is welcome. While sitting in the seat of consciousness, carry no opinion or judgment of what your partner is saying. Give them permission to be exactly as they are.

After your partner responds, refrain from reacting to what they say with nods, words, or even facial expressions. Instead, remain neutral, pause, and allow space and silence for your partner's expression to be heard and felt. After a few steady breaths, ask again, "What are you experiencing now?" The partner shares another, often deeper layer of their present-moment experience. After giving them time and space to answer, pause again and ask a third time, "What are you experiencing now?" Once more, while remaining in the seat of consciousness, listen without reacting, analyzing, comparing, or judging. Your partner's experience is what it is.

Thank your mitra for their participation. Then, switch roles.

When I did this, I had a life-changing encounter. I was incredibly moved by my partner's presence. The Vedic teacher Sri Nisargadatta

Maharaj said that the neutrality of consciousness "will blossom into an all-pervading and all-embracing love." This was my experience. My partner was neutral as I answered the questions, and I felt that neutrality as unconditional love. I could feel that she was fully present with me, distracted by nothing. Her energy conveyed that whatever I said was welcome. The space was open, free from anyone else's ideas, opinions, or judgments. There was no one telling me how to be, shaming me for saying or feeling something "wrong," or affirming that what I said was acceptable. After decades of trying to mold myself to the cultures and societies around me, on that day, in that moment, I allowed myself to truly be myself and speak honestly, without holding back.

Through this practice, I glimpsed the liberation of releasing the need for approval from cultures, societies, family, and friends. I remembered that I am allowed to trust myself, reconnect with my spirit, express it authentically, and live guided by its wisdom. While cultures, societies, family, and friends can be beautiful in many ways, we can respectfully shape our own path when our spirit's expression differs.

The potency of practices such as WAYEN is why communication is one of the Yogi's Way's twelve pillars. In your notebook, journal about your experience of the WAYEN practice.

Yoga teaches us to live with integrity, embracing ourselves fully, without rejecting any aspect of our being.

The psychospiritual practices I learned from Lee Joseph are invaluable tools that help us live our yoga and experience the healing that arises from embracing our wholeness and aligning mind, body, and spirit. The Yogi's Way programs incorporate a variety of communication practices developed by Lee Joseph, alongside influential methods like Nonviolent Communication, created by clinical psychologist Marshall Rosenberg.

Science and spirituality complement each other in many ways.

This is one of them. Yoga connects us to a space that is expansive. Consciousness is a boundless dimension. I believe my ancestors would be happy for yogis and psychotherapists to collaborate and refine our techniques to heal ourselves and to help others heal themselves. Such humility and collaboration are integral to the Yogi's Way programs, retreats, and trainings. Since studying with Lee, I've collaborated with psychotherapists working with Internal Family Systems, somatic, gestalt, and other therapies. Bringing such alliance to our clients and students has been deeply enriching for everyone involved.

For those of you who work in mental health, consider how you can utilize teachings of consciousness in your practices. Lee trained his students and clients to sit in the seat of consciousness before diving into the many modalities he taught. What is your vision of bringing this dimension to your clients?

You don't need to have an answer right now. I invite you to be in the question as you continue reading, keeping your mind open and curious.

3. Deepen the Five-Minute Optimal Breath Practice

Since Week Two, we have been cultivating a daily habit of optimal breathing. Each morning, we dedicate five minutes to establishing slow, diaphragmatic breathing through the nose, keeping the spine straight. Striving for a rhythmic six-second inhalation and equal exhalation, we tune in to our body and follow a comfortable pace with no strain.

This week, we will expand upon this practice.

1. If you wake up feeling stressed or anxious, try extending the duration of your exhalations so that they are longer than your inhalations. For example, inhale for four counts and exhale for six counts. Find a ratio that feels comfortable,

allowing you to breathe without strain. When you exhale for longer than you inhale, it activates the parasympathetic nervous system, which is responsible for the body's rest and digest functions. This can decrease your heart rate, lower blood pressure, and trigger a greater relaxation response than an even inhalation and exhalation.

2. Once you've established your breath pattern, shift your awareness from your mind to your heart. Intentionally evoke a positive emotion within your heart space. This could be gratitude for the blessings in your life or love for a friend, family member, or pet. We don't have to rely on external circumstances to experience positive emotions. We have the power to cultivate them in the present moment.

Renowned scientist and five-time *New York Times* bestselling author Gregg Braden elucidates the profound health benefits derived from just three minutes of a practice such as the one described above. By redirecting our focus from the mind to the heart, slowing down the breath, and embracing positive emotions, we initiate a transformation in our body's chemistry.

This results in strengthened immune defenses, particularly enhancing SIgA, the primary antibody response in the mucous membranes of the digestive system, beginning in the mouth and surpassing the effects of many antibiotics. Moreover, this practice activates longevity enzymes and fosters the healing of telomeres with the awakening of the telomerase enzyme. This can lead to benefits such as slowed cellular aging, enhanced cellular health, reduced risk of age-related diseases, and improved overall health and longevity.

On a molecular level, this practice alleviates stress, including stress stemming from environmental pollutants, impurities in water, and heavy oils in food. In a mere three minutes, DHEA levels surge over 100 percent, serving as a precursor to steroid hormones in both male and female bodies without supplements or dietary alterations, while cortisol levels decrease by approximately 23 percent. These benefits endure for up to six hours.

Engaging in this practice daily also cultivates familiarity with residing in the heart space. This offers respite from the mind and helps us cultivate a connection between the heart and the quantum field of consciousness. The vast, timeless, infinite dimension of consciousness cannot be grasped by the intellect, but it can be experienced from the heart.

Week Four Daily Practice Sequence

How is your practice space? Be sure to maintain a clean and uncluttered practice area. Whether it is a room in your home or a place at the foot of your bed, make the space pleasant to be in so you look forward to your precious practice time every day. This is your opportunity to begin developing the qualities of a spiritual warrior: determination, will, honesty, courage, daring, discipline, focus, patience, and endurance.

You can now turn the five-minute Optimal Breath practice into a three-minute exercise. Since you are becoming more familiar with slow, deep nasal breathing, it will take you less time each morning to establish yourself in this breath. As you do, remember to bring your awareness to your heart and evoke a positive emotion such as gratitude or love.

Here's a great sequence for the practices you have learned so far:

1. Optimal Breath practice: three minutes at the beginning of the day
2. All-Day Yoga
3. Sun Salutations with chakra awareness: fifteen minutes
4. Witness Meditation: six minutes

5. Savasana: five minutes
6. Journaling: five to ten minutes
7. Klesha Trigger Log: five to ten minutes at the end of the day

Total daily practice time: approximately forty to fifty minutes

Week Four Mitra Meeting

You now have a daily forty- to fifty-minute practice that you will continue not just this week but for the duration of this program. With your mitras, commit to it.

Share your progress with your mitras. How often did you remind yourself to practice All-Day Yoga this week? Were you able to maintain slow, deep breathing through the nose on most days? How is it to meet yourself from the radically open and accepting space of the witness? During the week, did you meet anyone else or an aspect of your life from the seat of consciousness? What was your experience of the WAYEN practice? How does your daily practice make you feel?

Key Terms from Week Four

Consciousness: An underlying, unchanging reality that is infinite space and possibility.

Witness: An open, welcoming, nonjudgmental presence.

Shravan: Listening.

Manan: Reflection.

Nididhyasana: Meditation for direct experience.

STORIES

Create an Empowering Narrative

What the mind dwells on, you become.

<small>UPANISHADS</small>

As mentioned in Week Two, one of the major kleshas is attachment. And one of our biggest attachments is to our own identities — the stories we tell ourselves about ourselves that end up
shaping our lives. This week we will investigate the labels and stories
that we identify with. We will explore how the way we define ourselves creates a story that either binds us or liberates us to explore
our potential.

The story you tell yourself becomes your reality.

<small>CHRIS HEMSWORTH</small>

When we place labels on ourselves, we tend to become them: I
am smart, I am dumb, I am healthy, I am broken, I am healing,
I am alone, I am connected. Our stories and labels are intricately intertwined with what we experience. For over three thousand years,
yogis have insisted that our mindset is everything. "What the mind
dwells on, you become," is a theme found in the Upanishads. Mystics
throughout the world agree. In the Dhammapada, the Buddha says,
"What we are today is a result of our thoughts from yesterday." The

Bible teaches, "As a man thinketh, so he is" (Proverbs 23:7). Now, neu-roscientists and physicists are discovering that what we think about, we bring about. Our thoughts become our reality. *Mind is matter.*

Jim is a student in our community who was struggling in life. After getting a divorce and losing his job, he'd been seeing himself as a victim. His story was that nothing ever worked out for him, he was wasting his life, and nothing would ever change. So often, he felt frustrated, angry, unhappy, and stuck. He projected his discontent onto all aspects of his life, creating and fortifying a prison of his own making. Jim couldn't believe how far he'd come from the healthy and thriving man he once was.

One day, Jim spoke with an old friend who told him what he needed to hear: that he had potential and that his attitude was dan-gerous and self-defeating. That same day Jim started to change his story. He began focusing his energy on improving his life. Instead of watching TV on the weekends, he joined a men's basketball team that met every Saturday and began to develop new friendships. He started eating more healthily and skipping his daily trip to the café near work to get a sweet treat. Instead of driving the three miles to his job, Jim began biking and enjoying time in nature. Soon, he decided to go back to school for a graduate degree.

Jim was changing the way he thought about himself. He was reconnecting with who he used to be — a person with dreams, aspi-rations, and vitality. He was determined to do the necessary work to rekindle that spirit and create a more fulfilling life.

Jim's shift in attitude set the stage for him to transform his life, and his story is a powerful reminder of how our beliefs shape our reality. The following teaching from Roopa Pai's commentary on the Brihadaranyaka Upanishad further illustrates the power of self-belief: A teacher gives two disciples an extremely challenging as-signment. The first disciple asks the teacher, "Do you really think I can accomplish this task?" The teacher turns the question around and asks the student: "Do you think you can?" The student replies, "No." The teacher says, "You have your answer."

The second student asks the same question. When the teacher asks this student, "Do you think you can?" the student says, "Yes." The teacher replies, "You have your answer."

This story teaches us: *When we believe we can, we do. When we believe we can't, we don't.*

Throughout history, we find people like Madam C. J. Walker, an African American woman who, in the late 1800s, overcame countless obstacles to create a business that helped other African American women. No one believed in Walker. Everyone laughed at her and labeled her inferior, including bankers she approached for loans and women she asked to become her partners in business. When one door closed, Walker knocked on others. She believed in herself and, against all odds, created a thriving business. Walker became the first female self-made millionaire in the United States during a time when women didn't even have the vote. Walker exemplified that accepting the stories other people construct about who we are is just as dangerous as creating our own limiting beliefs and identity.

My grandmother showed me by example that believing in our worthiness and capabilities enables us to cultivate a life filled with meaning, purpose, and joy even under daunting challenges. Born in a small town in central India, my grandmother entered an arranged marriage at the tender age of fourteen. She ended up raising her children on her own and confronted significant health issues. The adversities and societal obstacles she faced were formidable. Every day my grandmother filled her mind with mantras, affirmations that reminded her of her strength and capabilities. Her practice grounded her in her value and potential, and she approached life with confidence. Her daughters marvel at how much joy she infused their everyday lives with and what a warm, loving, and peaceful home she created for them.

During our adolescence, whenever my cousin Sonia and I would ask our grandmother about her hardships, she would respond to our indignation over her early marriage to a stranger with a smile and say, "That's just how things were." There was no bitterness in her voice. Instead, she exuded a firm belief in her own resilience and ability to face life with exuberance. My grandmother continues to teach me that we can strive to reform oppressive systems while making the most of our current circumstances. No matter what, joy is our birthright, and no one can take that away from us. When we intimately understand our true potential, the cards we've been dealt become less significant. What truly matters is how we play them, and that ultimately depends on our mindset.

Yoga helps us create that kind of mind — a mind that even under the most challenging circumstances finds purpose and thrives. Such a mind doesn't have to be rare. When life is oppressive, which it often is, the Upanishads and the Bhagavad Gita encourage us to dig deeper into our inner resources. Here, we find strength and creativity to rise above our challenges.

> *I lived in Auschwitz, and I can tell you that the greatest prison you will ever live inside is the prison you create in your own mind. Today, we have an opportunity to decide to hold on to hatred, or recognize that hatred is eating us up, to decide to be a survivor, instead of a victim of anyone or any circumstance. Auschwitz was an opportunity to discover my power within me.*
>
> DR. EDITH EVA EGER

We can think of a million reasons to feed the story of *I CAN'T*. Victim mentality is seductive to the ego. I've had moments while teaching yoga over the past twenty-three years when I've had the following thoughts: *It's too hard to make ends meet as a yoga instructor. It's easier for non-Indian people born into money to survive in this industry. It's easier for men to travel and teach and negotiate their rates and worth. It's harder as a woman and a single mother to run a business.* Et cetera.

I let these thoughts come and I let them go, always returning to my center, my spirit, my strength. This is what I've learned in life: I have the potential to move through the obstacles in front of me.

Rooted in my breath, I've learned how to ask for help while running a business — a lawyer to write contracts, an agent to take care of negotiations, clients to write testimonials, family to be with my daughter while I work, a coach to help me navigate the endless challenges that come with entrepreneurship. All of this has required being vulnerable, showing courage, taking financial risks, and stepping well beyond my comfort zone.

We may have a hundred examples of how the world is against us, and we could indeed be correct. But then what? We persist. The Bhagavad Gita teaches us to let obstacles, defeat, and disappointment guide us inward, tapping into the well of insight and strength that resides within. When we touch the deepest and most limitless parts of ourselves, we connect with the vast expanse of consciousness. In this space, we can rest, restore, strengthen, and allow room for fresh energy and insight to emerge. Here, creative energies rise, and we begin to see fresh and innovative solutions to the challenges in front of us.

One way to connect with the open and boundless space of consciousness is to understand what we are not.

Neti neti. "I am not this. I am not that."

> *I've let go of so much, the graveyards must be full*
> *of all the people I used to be.*
>
> Anonymous

When turning our gaze inward, we can identify the labels and identities that limit our lives and let them go, one by one. We come to the truth of our essential, boundless Self through a process of negating the labels.

The Brihadaranyaka Upanishad explains the ultimate truth of who we are as neti neti, "not this, not that." *I am not this, and I am not that.*

Any label placed on us is temporary and not entirely true. I can be kind in the morning and cruel in the afternoon. I can be alone today and choose to connect with community tomorrow. I can be vibrant and outgoing today and need to rest and retreat tomorrow. The Upanishads describe our true Self as devoid of any fixed quality or characteristic. We appear to be solid, but we are mostly empty space.

Quantum physicists describe a similar phenomenon: Nothing exists as it appears. We are made up of cells. Cells are made up of molecules. Molecules are made of atoms. Atoms are 99.9 percent empty space. A table, a person, and the earth all appear solid, but they're not. Solidity is an illusion. The truth, according to quantum physicists, is that every object and person is a field of pure potentiality. We are not fixed beings.

Here's the catch: Because we are nothing, we can be anything.

This isn't to say that I can close my eyes and become a bird. But I can grow up in poverty and learn how to build wealth. We can overcome the limits imposed by others, society, or our own internalized beliefs. Of course, it's essential that we put in the effort to make the changes we want to experience, as we are doing in this course.

To be present with the dimension of spaciousness or consciousness within us is one of the most powerful things we can do, because it is here that we directly experience our boundless potential. It is here that we ultimately connect with our creative energy and find moments of revelation that guide us on our path. Whatever we gain or lose in life, the space of pure potentiality at the core of our being remains unchanging. This sanctuary, this quiet field of infinite possibility, is always available to us. Our personality is a story we come up with that naturally changes. We don't have to become attached to it.

After having a child, I kept wondering when I would go back to feeling like my "normal" self again — the Reema I was before having a baby. I waited and wondered. I felt nostalgic and frustrated. Then, one day, I realized that Reema was gone. The Reema who remained was different, changed.

My practice was no longer one of trying to retrieve who I was before having a baby; rather, it was about being receptive to who I now was. Instead of this effort being depressing, it became exciting. Instead of holding on to a personality that no longer existed, I felt like a child discovering who I am.

The old parts of me were like fire or wind — I let them burn and be gone. I leaned into a deeper truth: I am space, a field of immeasurable possibility. I let myself rest and breathe here, allowing room for the new eventually to emerge.

The Bhagavad Gita encourages us to discover and live the truth of our innermost existence, rather than conform to external standards. When our outer life reflects our inner being, we grow into freedom where our integrity is not compromised. We live, not by submitting to outer authority or to the past, but by practicing the discipline of listening inwardly in the now.

In our achievement-oriented society, we are trained to do, do, do, create, create, create, and become, become, become. Vedic teachings remind us of how powerful it is to pause and let ourselves relax in the unknown. We may not know what is next in our life. Our body and mind might need to completely rest, restore, and be in the field of possibility. It's powerful to lean into the unknown and let the uncertainty be. Insight and creativity come to us when the mind and body are relaxed. It is a practice that is perhaps foreign to the modern world: to be OK in the not knowing. From the field of consciousness, we can receive energy and love that is deeply restorative, healing, and insightful. Only we can give ourselves permission to pause in silence and spacious presence. It is more than OK to be in the space between destruction and creation, the old and the new, dissolution and rebirth. To rest and breathe in the space that precedes creation is potent. For those of us living fast-paced lives, it is essential.

In My Own Hands

When I was growing up, my mother taught me a morning practice in which we sang a mantra while looking at the palms of our hands (see figure 9). The practice of reciting the mantra out loud or internally takes about fifteen seconds. The meaning of the mantra is: "I look to the tips of my fingers, where abundance resides. I look to the center of my hands, where there is wisdom and creativity. I look to the base of my hands, which represents perseverance. I acknowledge these qualities that reside in my own hands."

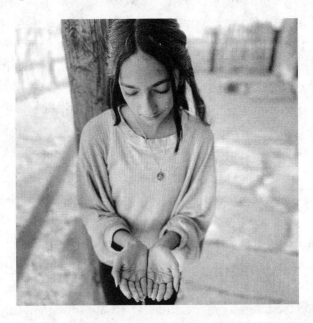

FIGURE 9: My daughter, Mila, practicing In My Own Hands.

Here is the mantra in Sanskrit:

कराग्रे वसते लक्ष्मीः करमध्ये सरस्वती ।
करमूले तु गोविन्दः प्रभाते करदर्शनम् ॥

Karagre Vasate Lakshmi Karamadhye Sarasvati
Karamule tu Govinda Prabhate Karadarshanam

In this way, we began each morning recognizing that our destiny lies in our hands rather than what the outer world gives to or takes from us. We approach the day with a sense of personal power, possibility, and positivity: *Whatever happens on this day, abundance, creativity, and perseverance live within me. It is up to me to recognize and use my inner resources.*

For the yogi, our story is simple. It has two main components:

1. I AM...pure potential. I am worthy, abundant, creative, and capable.
2. I CAN...overcome my obstacles, experience my full capacity, and give of myself completely and authentically.

So many of the mantras in the yoga tradition help us establish and embody this simple and empowering story: I can. I am capable, strong, and pure. Even if we don't know the details of our new story, we can rest in these ultimate truths that provide the backbone for our new narrative. Taking on these ultimate truths like a mantra, we can relax our mind. In an open and grounded mind, clarity and vitality are born. A popular anecdote suggests that Albert Einstein had some of his most profound insights while resting in his bathtub. As we grow up, the outer world, especially the media, often succeeds in convincing us that we need so many things to be complete: Not until I get that job, house, relationship, money, vacation will I be happy. It is a story we get so attached to that it clouds the wisdom we were born with and that we embraced so easily as children. It is only in the awakening to our own creativity, potential, and purpose that we experience real and lasting joy.

Only we can do the inner work of clearing the blocks to our true potential. The irony of the path is that we are not meant to do the work alone. We need support. Our mitras are our inner circle of closest companions. From that foundation, the circle expands. It may include a therapist who helps us to move through trauma, a support group that helps us overcome an addiction, a teacher who helps us develop a skill related to our svadharma, a nutritionist who helps us discover what foods and herbs are most suitable for our constitution, or a yogi who guides us in refining our techniques as we practice to release our granthis.

Asking for Help

Before becoming a mother, I thought success meant being able to do everything on my own. This belief was imprinted in me during the days I lived in New York City, working from nine to five. I felt the need to prove to myself and to the world that I could manage all aspects of life by myself. This only left me lonely and exhausted. The popular saying "It takes a village" is true.

If you're like me, you may hesitate to ask for help. I have found it can take time to locate our mitras and our community, but once we surround ourselves with the right people for us, they are happy to help, especially when they see someone trying to help themselves. What is more joyful than being able to help each other inch toward our svadharma? When each of us is thriving and giving our gifts, the net that holds us all strengthens.

I've shifted my narrative from being fiercely independent, capable of doing everything myself, to one where I ask for help when needed. This new narrative embraces our interconnectedness and the mutual support we provide each other. At times, I find myself in the role of Arjuna, overwhelmed by a klesha and needing support. Other times, I embody Krishna, sharing eternal truths and wisdom to help others. This new narrative encourages more honesty, vulnerability, and flexibility, allowing my roles to change as circumstances require.

Mantra

The Sanskrit word *mantra* comes from the root *man*, which means "mind," and the root *trā*, meaning "to protect" or "to liberate." A mantra literally protects and liberates us from our own mind. Since the stories we tell ourselves about ourselves shape our lives — either confining or freeing us — we replace destructive labels with mantras or affirmations that contribute to our well-being.

Some examples of mantras, which can serve as affirmations to reinforce an empowering story, include:

- *So ham:* "I am that," meaning, "I am consciousness, infinite possibility."
- I am capable and strong.
- I am present and powerful.
- I am worthy.
- I am supported.
- I am changing my thoughts and life.
- I am discovering and refining my gifts and purpose.
- I CAN.
- I am boundless potential.
- I am healing.
- I can thrive.
- I can rest, restore, and strengthen.

Week Five Practices

1. Work with Mantra

Read the mantras in the list above. Choose three that resonate with you right now. Write each of them three times in your notebook. Mantras introduce a constructive thought, which can replace a destructive one. A positive thought or memory induces a completely different biochemical reaction in the body than a negative one. Including mantras in our lives can alter our psychophysiology, releasing us from stress. Mantras help us develop a new habit of thinking, which ultimately influences our actions and realities. Every day this week, write these three mantras in your notebook three times each.

2. Breathe with the So Ham Mantra

In Week Two, you received the All-Day Yoga practice — to breathe slowly through the nose throughout the day. This week, when you feel yourself getting triggered, upset, or stressed for any reason, mentally chant *so* with the inhale and *ham* with the exhale (pronounced like "hum"). Do this for a minimum of three breaths. Ancient yogis identified *so ham* as the natural sound vibration of the breath. *So* is the inhalation. *Ham* is the exhalation.

This mantra is translated in two ways.

So comes from the root verb *sa*, which means "to be" or "to have power." The inhalation *so* infuses us with inspiration and a sense of personal power. The root verb *ham* means "to cast out, expel, exhale, or abandon." With every exhale, carry the intention to release something within you that doesn't serve you, such as a harmful thought or belief.

The Sanskrit root *saha*, from which *so* derives, means "that." *Ham* comes from the Sanskrit word *aham*, which means "I am." *So ham* also translates to "I am that." "That" refers to consciousness — the boundless field of pure potentiality. Again, when you are feeling stressed or triggered for any reason, try breathing with the so ham mantra for at least three breaths. Allow the mind to settle before reacting. *I am that field of possibility.* Inhale, breathe in inspiration. Exhale, relax into the spaciousness of your true Self.

3. Release Your Labels

Consider the two lists below. The first contains labels that describe patterns and habits we may identify with and get attached to. The second describes labels that may become roles in life. Using these lists as prompts, in your notebook write down the labels that you identify with and would like to release.

Patterns and Habits

Anger

Apathy

Argumentativeness

Arrogance

Believing "Appearance is everything"

Believing "Money is everything"

Believing "Money is evil"

Bossiness

Comparing self to others

Controlling

Dependence

Fear of change

Fear of confrontation

Fear of failure

Fear of intimacy

Fear of poverty

Fear of success

Feeling guilty

Feeling helpless

Feeling trapped

Feeling unworthy

Feeling withdrawn

Indecision

Independence

Intimidation

Needing to feel special

Needing to please

Needing to spend money to feel good

Optimism

Passivity

Perfectionism

Pessimism

Sarcasm

Self-obsession

Self-righteousness

Shutting down

Vengefulness

Victimhood

Workaholism

Worry

Roles

Angry one

Baby

Burden

Clown

Complainer

Damaged one

Disappointed one

Dreamer

Failure

Fighter

Genius

Hero

Loser

Misfit

Peacemaker

Perfect one

Princess

Rebel

Rescuer

Scapegoat

Sensitive one

Sick one

Slob

Special one

Spoiled one

Star

Success

Sufferer

Teacher

Troublemaker

Victim

Wild one

4. Examine Your Story

Whatever follows "I AM..." comes looking for you.

JOEL OSTEEN

The stories we tell ourselves about ourselves run our lives. When we change the narrative, we change our life. For example, if you tend to be a pleaser, you may feel guilty each time you say no to a request.

Your new story can be that you honor your body's signals and say no when your body says no. By doing so, you become a strong, authentic person who takes care of themselves as well as others. You begin to believe that when you say no, you are not a bad person. In fact, you are mending a deep wound and starting to create a new neural pathway in your brain that heals and liberates you and those around you.

Here's another example: You've labeled yourself as "the perfect one." Your new story is that you will share more of yourself even if your expressions are flawed. You will remind yourself that your imperfections make you human and relatable. Letting yourself be seen and heard even if you stumble gives others permission to express themselves even if their words don't flow perfectly.

One more example is that you carry a label of "clown." Whenever you go out, you feel people expect you to be the funny one, because this is how you usually are. Sometimes, when you're not feeling comical, this causes you anxiety. Instead of trying to meet these perceived expectations, your new story can be one of letting your friends see other sides of who you are.

In your journal, write a story about who you have been and the labels and roles that have shaped your mind and reality. Include where some of these labels came from. Reflect on which of these labels no longer serves you.

5. Do a Fire Ceremony

In Sanskrit, a ceremony is called a *puja*, meaning "reverence" or "honor." Pujas, which are central to Vedic practices, can range from simple to elaborate. In a fire puja, the fire symbolizes purification and transformation. Seekers put various offerings into the fire, accompanied by prayers, to ask for purification, protection, blessings, and guidance. These rituals are considered powerful, bringing about spiritual cleansing and positive change.

This week, try performing a simple fire ceremony to help you release the old stories that are holding you back. If your mitras live near you, get together with them to do this ceremony. Otherwise, do it on your own and let your mitras know about your experience in this week's meeting.

On individual pieces of paper, write down the labels and stories that you are ready to let go of. You will be making a fire in a fireplace at home or in an outdoor firepit. Clean the space where you will make the fire. Just as with your practice space, make it free of clutter. Take a shower or bath and put on fresh, comfortable clothes. Make sure you are well hydrated and not too hungry or too full so you can focus on the ceremony.

To begin the ceremony, light your fire. Call in your guides, as we did in Week One, and review your motivation. Express your intention to remove blocks within yourself so you can experience your full potential and contribute the gifts you were born to share. Offer the pieces of paper with the labels and stories written on them to the fire. As you do, you can either recite (internally or out loud) one of the mantras you selected in the first exercise this week (page 111) or create a personal prayer in your own words — for example, "I release the labels that don't serve me and make room for what truly does."

When you acknowledge the stories that limit you and then give them away, their hold on you diminishes. As the papers burn, visualize your mind releasing its grip on these identities. As the grip loosens, notice if space begins to open within you. Relax your mind and breathe into this space.

Consider how some of your life challenges have made you stronger and wiser today. Close your ceremony with a sense of gratitude.

i am not a victim of my life
what I went through
pulled a warrior out of me
and it is my greatest honor to be her

RUPI KAUR

6. Space Meditation

Practice the five-minute Space Meditation below every day this week, gradually becoming more familiar with the spaciousness that lies at your center. The best time to practice is in the early morning after a cup of tea and before the people you live with wake up (if you don't live alone). The next best time to practice is in the early evening as you wind down from your day, preferably before dinner.

Space Meditation

Take a comfortable, meditative seat and set your timer for five min-
utes. Close your eyes and begin to see yourself as empty of qualities and
characteristics, especially the ones you released in the fire ceremony. Re-
member, science has shown that we are 99.9 percent empty space. This is
in line with the Vedic teaching that our true nature is infinitely spacious
and expansive — devoid of any fixed quality or characteristic.

Breathe into the openness that lies at the center of your being.
Lean into it. Relax. Resist the temptation to replace old identities with
new ones. How does it feel to identify more with the openness than
any quality or characteristic? Let your mind rest and experience the
spaciousness. Be like a detective — immerse yourself in this openness
completely.

When you practice this five-minute meditation, keep your mind relaxed and focused. Most importantly, resist the temptation to replace old labels with new ones. How does it feel to let yourself be empty and open? Is there a freedom to be experienced right here and now?

> *Create a clearing in the dense forest of your life*
> *and wait there patiently.*
>
> MARTHA POSTLETHWAITE, "Clearing"

On the last day of the week, before your weekly meeting with your mitras, practice this five-minute meditation. Then, complete the following sentences in your journal:

- When I let myself breathe and relax into the openness at the core of my being, I feel…
- In the past, I've been in the habit of thinking and saying to myself: *I AM…*
- I'm creating a new habit of thinking and saying to myself: *I AM…*

The new thought habit can be: *I am open, I am letting go of labels that don't serve me, I am learning to accept uncertainty, I am worthy of love, I am pure potential, I am letting myself relax in the space that precedes creation*, or anything else that resonates with you. Recognizing and letting go of labels and identities that you may have been holding on to for years and even decades is powerful. To allow yourself to breathe into the openness that you have cultivated is even more potent. There's no rush to fill in that space.

7. In My Own Hands

When you wake up in the morning, before your feet even touch the ground, take fifteen seconds to look at the palms of your hands. Say to yourself, *Abundance lies at my fingertips, creativity and wisdom in the center of my hands, and perseverance at their base. It's up to me to draw upon my inner resources.* Alternatively, you can simplify by looking at the palm of your hands and mentally saying, *Abundance, creativity, wisdom, and perseverance lie in my own hands. Today, I will draw upon my inner resources.*

If you are interested, learn the Sanskrit mantra and recite it as is described on page 109. You can listen to the mantra at TheYogisWay .com/thebook.

Week Five Daily Practice Sequence

Here's a suggested sequence for the practices you have learned so far:

1. In My Own Hands: fifteen seconds (when you wake up)
2. Optimal Breath practice: three minutes at the beginning of the day
3. All-Day Yoga
4. Sun Salutations with chakra awareness: fifteen minutes
5. Witness Meditation: six minutes
6. Space Meditation: five minutes
7. Savasana: five minutes
8. Journaling: five to ten minutes
9. Klesha Trigger Log: five to ten minutes at the end of the day

Total daily practice time: approximately forty-five to fifty-five minutes

I create my way
I paint out my days
I create my story
I create my glory

ALEXIA CHELLUN, "Just before I Sleep"

Week Five Mitra Meeting

In your meeting with your mitras, discuss this week's practices. What did you experience? Breakthroughs? Breakdowns? Questions? Speak without holding back, carrying tenderness and compassion for yourself. Listen without judgment, holding affection for your mitras. There is a power in connection and honesty that is difficult to describe but that each of us can experience when we are willing. Remember, magic happens outside of our comfort zone.

Key Terms from Week Five

Mantra: A word, sound, or phrase that protects and liberates you from your own mind.

Neti neti: "I am not this. I am not that."

Puja: Ceremony.

So ham: "I am that"; "I am consciousness — infinite light and possibility."

MANTRA

Protect and Liberate Your Mind

The mind binds us or frees us.

AMRITABINDU UPANISHAD (2.1)

I n Week Five, we released some of the stories and identities that limit us and began to get comfortable in the space of pure potential that lies at our center. This week, using a series of mantras, we will begin to plant seeds in this space that cultivate confidence, along with a sense of personal power and agency, helping to overcome the kleshas of doubt, fear, shame, and low self-worth.

I don't know anyone who hasn't struggled with self-doubt. At some point or another, most of us have felt that we aren't good enough. *Who am I to be this person, embody that role, have that job?* we wonder. Even if we succeed, we may experience impostor syndrome, a persistent inability to believe that our skills and efforts are the real reason for our success. *Do I truly have something valuable to contribute?* we may ask ourselves. Like all thoughts, words, and stories, we can change this one too. Instead of saying to ourselves, *I'm not good enough* or *I can't*, we say, *Why not me?*

Cultivating Confidence and Self-Worth

The neural pathways that carry thoughts and stories of self-doubt often run deep. It takes time, effort, and discipline to create new pathways that represent a story of faith in ourselves. We each carry the same amount of light and possibility within us. Yoga is a journey of self-discovery that entails recognizing this light and potential.

Psychologists report that the leading negative personal perceptions in our society today are low self-esteem, shame, and self-loathing. Social media is contributing to mental health crises, harming the minds of youth and adults. In October 2023, forty-one states and the District of Columbia brought a lawsuit against tech giant Meta for promoting addictive social media features to minors. New Jersey Attorney General Matt Platkin stated, "Children are spending hours upon hours scrolling and being subjected to images and words that exacerbate a number of health and social issues including body image, eating disorders, anxiety, loneliness, depression, and envy."

The first step to transformation is allowing yourself to feel the pain of self-loathing, self-doubt, and shame. Whether only a trace of any of these emotions lives within you or one of them plays a strong role in your life, breathe deeply when they arise. Acknowledge them, and hold them with compassion and tenderness, as you would hold a small child. Give yourself permission to experience the emotion fully. Be brave. Step into the fire and feel the depth of it. When you let yourself experience it without judgment or guilt — which serve no purpose — the emotion becomes a door to something different. When you make peace with an emotion that is a natural part of the human experience, letting yourself feel it without fighting, judging, or resisting, a space is born. As we accept ourselves fully, we open ourselves to experience the broad range of emotions, including hope, wonder, self-love, and a sense of potential. It is in the complete acceptance of what is present that we merge into the field of possibility, which is the deepest reality of consciousness.

This week, we will learn the twelve classic Sun Salutation mantras. Each mantra is an affirmation that helps us cultivate confidence and a positive narrative about ourselves, feeding the stories "I CAN" and "Why Not Me?" Through this traditional practice, we begin our day by reminding ourselves of our value and potential. In Week Eight, we will begin to incorporate the mantras into our twelve-step Sun Salutation movement sequence. Through a practice of movement accompanied by mantra, we will cultivate a sense of personal power while also improving our body image and decreasing feelings of anxiety, sorrow, and jealousy. When our Sun Salutation practice incorporates movement, breathing, mantra, subtle body awareness, contemplation, meditation, and deep rest, it becomes a complete practice in itself.

Surya Namaskara has its roots in the Rigveda, which contains mantras that offer deep gratitude to the sun for the energy it bestows on all life. Adoration of the sun and practices to receive and assimilate the sun's primal energy are traditions shared by ancient indigenous communities worldwide, including the Egyptians, Greeks, Native Americans, and Chinese, as well as the Aztec, Inca, and Maya civilizations. In India, asana, or yoga postures, were added years after the mantras extolling the sun were written in the Vedas. As our modern lifestyles have become increasingly more sedentary, these postures are more important than ever.

The twelve mantras acknowledge twelve aspects of the sun's light that also live within us. By recognizing and appreciating these qualities, we open ourselves to embody them, creating a positive and empowering environment within and around us. The movement opens the mind and body to receive the sun's energy. The mantras facilitate its transfer and assimilation. The process instills a sense of possibility and connection with our primary energy source. With ongoing practice, the body and mind become radiant like the sun.

Sanskrit mantras comprise sound vibrations designed to uplift the mind and free it of its harmful tendencies. Each of the twelve Sun Salutation mantras include *Om* and *Namah*. *Om* is the universal vibration. It is the essence of ultimate reality, signifying the infinite that underlies creation, preservation, and dissolution. *Namah* means "bow" or "salutation," expressing deep reverence, respect, and surrender. It is often used in mantras to honor and connect with the sacred, both within and beyond.

Mantras can be recited out loud, whispered, or repeated silently in one's mind. Practicing mantra is a powerful way to replace negative thought patterns that drain our vitality with sounds that are energizing, empowering, and liberating. Let's become familiar with the Sun Salutation mantras.

The Twelve Sun Salutation Mantras

To hear the pronunciation of each mantra, visit TheYogisWay.com /thebook.

1. ***Om Mitraya Namah:* "Salutation to the one who is a friend to all."** As we learned in Week One, *mitra* is the Sanskrit word for "friend." The sun is the universal friend who gives light, heat, and energy to all beings equally, without discrimination. Sometimes the one we need to be the most affectionate toward is ourself. As we offer deep gratitude to the sun for being a universal friend, we acknowledge and awaken our own potential to be a friend to ourselves and others.

2. ***Om Ravaye Namah:* "Salutation to the shining one who bestows radiance and blessings and is the cause for change."** As we receive the radiance of the sun with gratitude, we

recognize and ignite our own capacity to become a cause for change and a blessing to our surroundings.

3. *Om Suryaye Namah:* **"Salutation to the one who initiates action."** As we honor the sun's dynamic energy that fuels action, we acknowledge and reflect on our own ability to initiate meaningful activity in the world — in both material and subtle planes of existence.

4. *Om Bhanave Namah:* **"Salutation to the one who spreads light and illumines."** As we recognize how each dawn dispels the darkness of night and a teacher helps remove confusion from one's mind, we recognize and awaken our ability to illuminate our mind and the minds of those around us through our words, actions, and intentions. A simple smile, a kind word, or a hug can have a profound impact.

5. *Om Khagaye Namah:* **"Salutation to the one who moves through the sky."** As we appreciate the sun's daily journey across the sky, we reflect on and activate our own ability to move through our obstacles with energy and grace.

6. *Om Pushne Namah:* **"Salutation to the source of strength and nourishment (mental, physical, and spiritual)."** As we gratefully receive the sun's nourishing energy, we awaken our own capacity to bring nourishment to ourselves and to the earth, people, animals, and other beings that surround us.

7. *Om Hiranyagarbhaya Namah:* **"Salutation to the golden healing light that contains everything and helps awaken creativity."** As we respectfully receive the sun's healing, we recognize and bring forth our creative energy and become a healing influence.

8. *Om Marichaye Namah:* **"Salutation to the giver of light with infinite rays who helps us discern what is real versus illusion."** As we give thanks for that aspect of the sun's light

that helps us discern between what is real and unreal, we acknowledge and unleash our own ability to express truth in our lives.

9. *Om Adityaya Namah:* **"Salutation to the cosmic mother, whose light lives within us all."** We recognize the light in all beings and bring forth our ability to treat ourselves and each other with respect and understanding.

10. *Om Savitre Namah:* **"Salutation to the stimulating power of the sun, which produces everything and is responsible for life."** Savitre is said to represent the sun before rising. The stimulating and arousing qualities of Savitre bring us into the waking state of activity that ultimately produces everything and is responsible for life. As we pay respect to the sun's creative power, we recognize our responsibility and capacity to be a creator in our own lives.

11. *Om Arkaya Namah:* **"Salutation to the one who removes afflictions and is worthy of praise and glory."** As we salute the sun's role in helping us heal, we acknowledge and commit to doing our part in overcoming afflictions of mind and body.

12. *Om Bhaskaraya Namah:* **"Salutation to the giver of wisdom and spiritual truth, lighting the way to liberation."** As we give thanks to and receive the sun's light, we awaken our potential to be a keeper and giver of liberating wisdom.

This week, spend about ten minutes each day reviewing these twelve mantras. Say the mantras out loud or silently. Contemplate the meaning of each mantra. Give thanks to the sun for what each mantra represents and visualize the qualities of each mantra awakening inside yourself. You will receive tremendous benefits from this alone. Remember your motivation. We practice yoga so we have more energy, love, and wisdom to give.

As you incorporate the twelve mantras into your daily routine, feel free to personalize them in a way that resonates with you. Also, if the Sanskrit terms feel overwhelming, you may replace them with short English translations, such as the ones given below. The Sanskrit language is powerful. Each syllable within the mantra holds the energy of the aspect of the sun it represents. Still, if Sanskrit is completely new to you, take your time to bring it into your practice.

For easy reference, here are brief translations of each mantra:

1. *Om Mitraya Namah:* "Friendly and affectionate to all"
2. *Om Ravaye Namah:* "Cause for change"
3. *Om Suryaye Namah:* "Inspires action"
4. *Om Bhanave Namah:* "Diffuses light"
5. *Om Khagaye Namah:* "Moves through obstacles"
6. *Om Pushne Namah:* "Nourishes oneself and others"
7. *Om Hiranyagarbhaya Namah:* "Brings healing"
8. *Om Marichaye Namah:* "Discerns truth from illusion"
9. *Om Adityaya Namah:* "Respect to the cosmic mother, whose light lives within all"
10. *Om Savitre Namah:* "Creates everything, responsible for life"
11. *Om Arkaya Namah:* "Removes afflictions, is worthy of praise"
12. *Om Bhaskaraya Namah:* "Illumines liberating wisdom"

As I mentioned earlier in this chapter, after we've had two weeks to become familiar with the depth and significance of each mantra, in Week Eight we will begin to incorporate the mantras into our twelve-step Surya Namaskara movement practice. We will be using every major muscle group in the body and our breath in a certain way while planting powerful seeds in the mind with each mantra. The masters created the practice this way for a reason. As we exert the effort to do something productive and healthy, we are identifying the attributes within us that we aspire to embody fully.

Vedic texts continually encourage us with reminders of the light and potential that are our essence. The Bible echoes this sentiment: "You are the light of the world" (Matthew 5:14). The Brihadaranyaka Upanishad explains that the individual is inseparable from the universal, like a wave and an ocean. Not only are the waves and ocean inseparable from one another, they are made of the same essence: water. In the same way, each of us is made of the same limitless potential as the Universe and are inseparable from it.

> *Think of the power of the Universe…turning the Earth, growing trees. That's the same power within you…if you'll only have the courage and the will to use it.*

> CHARLIE CHAPLIN

To have the intellectual knowledge that we are pure potential is an important beginning, but it's not enough, even if quantum physicists have proved this. To experience this truth directly — and to embody it — is entirely different. This takes daily disciplined practice. It takes a rewiring of the brain to disable the messages it may have received for decades — *I can't, It's impossible, I'm not good enough.* The power of tapping into and nurturing our inner light and creative potential may be something new. Engaging in daily practice sets us up to experience this.

As we learned last week, we are empty of any fixed quality or characteristic. We experience life on the basis of the impressions in our mind. The Bhagavad Gita states: "What the mind dwells on, you experience." In this fertile ground that is our life and our essence, why not plant seeds of personal power, creativity, love, wisdom, and abundance? This is what we do by reciting the mantras above. No one and nothing can give us these qualities, but we can cultivate them within our own mind through practice.

Yoga is a sacred discipline in which we create our life from the inside out. As we ignite the power of our mind, we become the master gardener, actively shaping our life through our thoughts. We intentionally plant seeds in our mind for what we want to experience in our life. If we don't truly believe that we are worthy of receiving life's greatest gifts, this doubt becomes an obstacle to creating our best life.

Surya Namaskara mantras help you cultivate the confidence and worthiness that are foundational on the path. Remember, you mustn't believe anything blindly. Practice and see what unfolds in your own life. It takes focus, discipline, determination, and will to practice daily. You have accountability partners. You are not on your own. Continue to cultivate these qualities of a spiritual warrior with your mitras.

Scientific research has confirmed that self-affirmations work. They have been shown to improve self-esteem, promote better health, enhance academic and professional performance, and reduce stress and resistance to change. Studies indicate that individuals who regularly engage in positive affirmations report lower levels of depression, decreased incidence of suicidal thoughts, reduced substance abuse, and alleviated anxiety. Through consistent repetition, positive statements can rewire the brain, instilling belief in oneself and inspiring corresponding actions.

Embrace the power of positive self-talk and enjoy its integration into your daily life, starting with this week's practices.

Week Six Practices

1. New Thoughts, New Patterns

This week, take about ten minutes every day to review the meanings of the twelve Surya Namaskara mantras (page 124). As you do this daily, new pathways are being created in the mind. Which thought patterns that were formed in childhood or adulthood are you releasing? How does it feel to replace them with the support of these mantras? Journal about your experience. Here are some questions you can ask yourself as prompts, as well as examples of possible answers. After answering each question, take a moment to visualize yourself embodying your response.

1. *Om Mitraya Namah:* **How can I be more affectionate and kind to myself and others?** For example, you might write: "Instead of beating myself up when I make a mistake, I'm going to practice intelligent regret. I will acknowledge the mistake, regret it, learn from it, forgive myself, apologize to someone if needed, and do my best not to do it again."

2. *Om Ravaye Namah:* **What do I want to change?** For example: "I want to be more present with my child. I will make the effort to stay away from my devices when we are together."

3. *Om Suryaye Namah:* **What action do I want to inspire?** For example: "I want to be so relaxed and trusting of life that I inspire others to relax and trust life, too."

4. *Om Bhanave Namah:* **What is one way I see myself spreading my light?** For example: "I want to cook healthy meals for friends and family," or "I want to let people know more often when I appreciate them." Remember to take a moment to close your eyes and envision yourself shining in this way.

5. *Om Khagaye Namah:* **What obstacles am I facing right now?** For example: "It's been hard to make it to the gym and take care of myself by exercising. I will think of my healthy, active friends and let them inspire me."

6. *Om Pushne Namah:* **What is one way I can nourish myself and someone else this week?** For example: "I want

to drink more water and eat less sugar. I'm going to buy my daughter a fun water bottle, so she is inspired to drink more water, too."

7. *Om Hiranyagarbhaya Namah:* **How do I want to bring healing to myself or another?** For example: "I want to share my poetry with those I feel it can help."

8. *Om Marichaye Namah:* **How can I illumine truth?** For example: "I will start with letting my friend know how I've been feeling hurt by her actions."

9. *Om Adityaya Namah:* **How can I pay respect to the cosmic mother and to the light that lives within us all?** For example: "I will spend time with people who I know have different views than me. I will foster understanding and unity rather than divisive thoughts."

10. *Om Savitre Namah:* **How can I take responsibility for something I'm creating in my life?** For example: "I've been feeling lonely, and I haven't made the effort to stay in touch with good friends."

11. *Om Arkaya Namah:* **How can I do my part in removing afflictions in my mind or body?** For example: "I can try to share more openly with my mitras in our weekly meetings."

12. *Om Bhaskaraya Namah:* **How can I spread liberating wisdom?** For example: "I can remind my best friend who has been struggling with self-worth that she is strong, capable, and full of potential. I can stay by her side and support her to follow through with some tough decisions that she's been wanting to make."

2. *Refine Your Breathing Practice*

How is your All-Day Yoga practice going? Remind yourself to do ADY by asking yourself these two questions throughout the day:

- Am I breathing through the nose?
- Can I lengthen my inhales and exhales?

Remember, you have the option to add the so ham mantra (page 112) to your breathing practice. Here are some additional questions that will help you nurture your ADY this week:

- How many times a day do I find myself remembering to shift from mouth breathing to nasal breathing? To slow down the breath?
- How does it feel to breathe deeply and slowly through the nose?
- How does it feel to breathe into the belly instead of the chest?
- A six-second inhale and six-second exhale is the ideal length, which we work up to. What rhythm feels comfortable for me now?

Week Six Daily Practice Sequence

1. In My Own Hands: fifteen seconds
2. Optimal Breath practice: three minutes at the beginning of the day
3. All-Day Yoga
4. Review the meanings of the twelve Sun Salutation mantras: ten minutes
5. Sun Salutations with chakra awareness: fifteen minutes
6. Witness Meditation: six minutes
7. Savasana: five minutes
8. Journaling: five to ten minutes
9. Klesha Trigger Log: five to ten minutes at the end of the day

Total daily practice time: approximately fifty to sixty minutes

Week Six Mitra Meeting

You are halfway through this course! Honor the wins and share the struggles of the past six weeks. How is the twelve-step Sun Salutation practice with chakra awareness that you learned in Week Three going? Are you comfortable in each pose? Do you need to modify the sequence in any way? Do you practice one breath per movement, or do you allow yourself a few breaths in each pose? What has been your experience with daily review of the twelve mantras introduced in this chapter? What do these mantras bring up for you? Are you feeling a shift from doubt to faith? From fear to trust?

End your mitra meeting today with a celebration.

Key Terms from Week Six

Om: Universal vibration, the infinite underlying all phenomena.

Namah: Bow, salutation, respectful acknowledgment made with humility and surrender.

CHOICES

*Become the Driver of the Mind
Instead of Its Passenger*

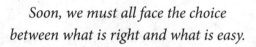

*Soon, we must all face the choice
between what is right and what is easy.*

J. K. ROWLING, *Harry Potter and the Goblet of Fire*

I n Week One, we developed our support network, our trusted inner circle with whom we can be transparent, vulnerable, and courageous. In Week Two, we understood that realizing our svadharma (purpose and potential) and reaching higher states of consciousness require an acknowledgment of our kleshas and a determination to understand and work through them. In Week Three, we began to learn how thoughts and emotions affect our health. In Week Four, we started to meet ourselves — both the pleasant and the painful aspects — from the open, welcoming, and nonjudgmental presence of witnessing consciousness.

In Week Five, we addressed one of the most powerful kleshas: attachment to the stories we identify with. We released labels that limit us, creating room within to rest, restore, and eventually bring forth something new. Last week, our sixth, we began to cultivate an empowering narrative about ourselves, graced with self-worth, confidence, and possibility. This week, we will explore more deeply the choices available to us to replace destructive and limiting thought patterns with ones that are liberating and empowering.

Through these practices, we are learning to become the driver of our mind instead of its slave. Ultimately, yoga teaches that *you are not your ever-changing mind and body. You are the Self who can operate the mind and body with wisdom.* We have too much love to give to let harmful thoughts destroy our health and destiny. It is a habit to tap into the field of pure potentiality that lives within. It is a practice to get familiar with it. It is a lifestyle to live in accordance with it.

If you're feeling overwhelmed or finding the journey challenging, know that most of us share the same experience. Engaging in spiritual practice — enlightening the mind and opening the heart — can be one of the toughest tasks we undertake in life. Embrace the journey, recognizing that progress is rarely linear. It's more like a spiral than a straight path. Challenges we believe we've overcome may resurface many times. In the second chapter of the Bhagavad Gita, Krishna understands Arjuna's struggle to absorb the profound wisdom and teachings and offers him reassurance, affirming, "On this path, effort never goes to waste, and there is no failure. Even a little effort towards spiritual awareness will protect you from the greatest fear" (2.40).

The Chosen One

One of the central themes of the Upanishads, as expressed in the Chandogya Upanishad (6.8.7), is the principle of *Tat Tvam Asi*: "You are that." You are the one who can let go of what no longer serves you and make room for the new. You are the one who can move through the obstacles in front of you and create a life of meaning and purpose. You are the one and only one who can change your thoughts and your life. You are it. The immeasurable light and potential of the Universe live inside you. Clear the blocks within. Know and honor who you truly are.

The Katha Upanishad explains that in every moment, we have a choice between two paths. One is easy and brings instant gratification to oneself. The other is difficult in the beginning but ends up bringing lasting benefit to all. These two paths have specific Sanskrit terms with no English parallel: *preya* (प्रेय) and *shreya* (श्रेय). Preya is pleasant in the moment but soon fades into the opposite (eating ice cream every day and then finding out you are diabetic). Shreya is often difficult in the moment, requiring courage and will (confronting your spouse with an uncomfortable topic), but it brings lasting benefit to all — healing, truth, peace, liberation. The wise choose the one that brings lasting joy, even though it requires patience and perseverance. Those led by impatience choose preya, mistakenly thinking they are wise.

We all want shreya (peace, health, freedom), but because that choice is often harder to make and requires bravery and daring, we tend to choose preya, the path that is easy, comfortable, and accepted.

For example, Jane had gained thirty pounds. She had heard of a great new exercise program being offered after work. She knew it was important to lose weight. It would give her more energy to extend to her family and friends. However, taking part in the exercise program would require coming home one hour later every evening, and she didn't want to miss her favorite TV show. She chose preya.

Chris was miserable in his job as a contractor. He had saved more than enough money to take a one-year sabbatical and pursue his dream of becoming a photographer. Chris had won many photography contests since he was a teenager. Yet being a full-time artist was unacceptable to his family. He was scared to challenge his family's fears and opinions and decided to stick with his job. Preya won.

I love making music. When I sing mantra or play the piano,

both I and the people around me feel a sense of peace. This has always been something precious and meaningful to me. I've told myself that every morning I will spend twenty minutes working on a song instead of getting distracted with *x*, *y*, and *z*. I still have a hard time keeping this commitment. So often preya wins.

It is a struggle to choose between what we know is beneficial for us but difficult in the moment (shreya) and what we know isn't so good for us but easier in the moment (preya). The issue often isn't that we don't know what to do. It's that we don't take action on what we know is best for us. Remember:

> Preya = pleasant now, can be harmful in the long term
> Shreya = difficult now, beneficial in the long term

Every moment holds an opportunity to exercise our freedom of choice, even in the most dire situations. When it may be easiest to simply give up, we can choose the more difficult but rewarding path: to persevere. After having everything stripped away from him, the Austrian psychiatrist and Holocaust survivor Viktor Frankl had the powerful realization that no one can take away his freedom to choose his thoughts and attitude. As a prisoner in concentration camps, Frankl witnessed unimaginable atrocities and experienced profound loss, including the deaths of his loved ones. Despite the harrowing conditions of the Holocaust, Frankl maintained a sense of inner resolve by focusing on his belief that every individual possesses the capacity to find meaning in their experiences, regardless of the circumstances. He saw his purpose as bearing witness to, and eventually documenting, the human capacity for resilience, courage, and dignity, even amid the horrors of genocide. He believed in the power of finding meaning and purpose as essential for human survival, resilience, and psychological well-being. In his seminal work *Man's Search for Meaning*, he shows us that even in the darkest of times, we can discover purpose and meaning, inspiring us all to persevere.

> *Everything can be taken from a man but one thing: the last of human freedoms — to choose one's attitude in any given set of circumstances, to choose one's own way.*
>
> VIKTOR E. FRANKL, *Man's Search for Meaning*

The Right Choice for You

The Bhagavad Gita describes how creating a life of integrity and purpose was never meant to be easy. We will stumble and fall a hundred times. We must keep getting up. We will be tempted to follow the path of others, but it's essential to stick with our own, no matter how much we struggle. Easier options will constantly lure us but will never bring us the satisfaction that the path of svadharma will — discovering, nurturing, and refining our unique gifts and destiny.

> *It is better to follow your own path and be clumsy than to perfectly follow another's.*
>
> BHAGAVAD GITA (3.35)

The Sanskrit word *dharma* means "right action, duty, or purpose." As we learned earlier, *svadharma* means "the right action for you in this moment." Whether your svadharma is to sit quietly in your room and write poetry, give attention to your child as a connected and present parent, study for an exam, or climb a mountain, one isn't better than another. Your svadharma is what it is. There is no right, wrong, better, or worse. Your svadharma is your unique creative energy in action, which is tied to the creative forces of the Universe.

The Individual Spirit is inseparable from Universal Energy.

BRIHADARANYAKA UPANISHAD (1.4.10)

We have an awareness within us that knows the best choice for us in each moment. However, these choices aren't always easy or familiar; they may require us to confront difficulties and navigate the unknown.

In our hectic lives, we often lose touch with our inner knowing. We may succumb to the voice of fear instead of heeding the deeper voice of our truth. The more we ignore our inner guidance, the quieter it becomes. Practices such as meditation and journaling help us develop our connection with this inner wisdom, fostering trust in ourselves and our inherent knowing.

If your path is different from the norms of the society and culture in which you live, it is especially hard to follow. However, when you take the first and often scary steps to honor your svadharma, the Universe moves mountains to support you, bringing the right people and opportunities into your life. To experience this, you must do your part, cultivating faith in the Universe through your own courage and experiences. As the popular saying goes, "Jump, and the net will appear."

When I left my career at the United Nations in New York City, I was terrified. I didn't have a job waiting for me. I didn't know how I would pay my bills and survive. I was confident that I would find a job but wasn't sure when or what it would be. It took several months for things to fall into place, and I did feel quite anxious during that time. Eventually, I walked into the yoga studio where I would be offered a full-time job with a set salary that covered my expenses. There, I learned about the yoga industry while making great friends and connecting with a community of kindred spirits. Since that moment in 2002, doors have continually opened, been left ajar, and closed. Through each trial, I've learned that the more I trust myself and open my mind, the more the world opens to me. Yoga has not made me fearless. But it has given me the courage to honor my svadharma and step through some of those open doors even in the face of trepidation.

> *The Other is the one who taught me what I should be like,*
> *but not what I am.... From the moment I ousted the Other*
> *from my life, the Divine Energy began to perform its miracles.*

> PAULO COELHO, *By the River Piedra I Sat Down and Wept*

To help us with the conundrum of choosing preya over shreya, the Katha Upanishad and Bhagavad Gita describe how to use our senses, impulses, intellect, and consciousness harmoniously by presenting an analogy of a chariot and driver (see figure 10). The allegories in these texts carry tremendous meaning, addressing the many tendencies of the human mind. The texts help us see how the mind can be our greatest enemy or our best friend, depending on how we approach it. If we befriend the mind and learn how to use it, it will empower us. Otherwise, it can lead to our downfall.

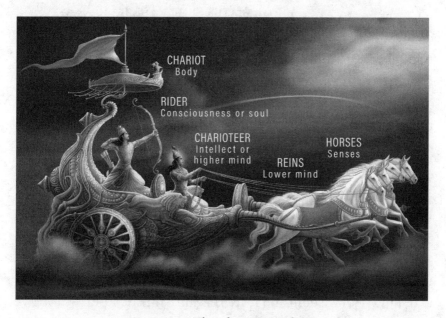

FIGURE 10: The chariot analogy.

The chariot represents our physical body. It is drawn by several horses, which symbolize the five senses (taste, smell, touch, hearing, vision) through which we relate to the external world. These five senses influence our emotions and can give rise to kleshas such as attachment or anger. Either the horses send us into a ditch or they carry us forward on a meaningful path of svadharma. The reins represent our lower mind, which is driven by impulses — the part of the mind that is conditioned and on autopilot. From here, the senses (horses) receive their instructions and act.

Krishna, the charioteer, stands in for the intellect, our higher mind, which has the capacity to distinguish between what is pleasant for us in the moment and what is beneficial for all in the long term. The higher mind sees clearly and keeps us from ending up in a ditch. You are the rider, the Self (consciousness or soul) who has the potential to listen to the higher mind and direct the body, impulses, emotions, and senses with wisdom and understanding.

For many of us, the horses go wherever they please, constantly chasing after preya (short-term pleasures) and leading us away from our true purpose and potential. The chariot (body) becomes worn down, the horses (senses) get bored, and the charioteer (higher mind) becomes dull. The rider (Self, consciousness, or soul) may be completely absent from the journey.

The solution is to train the charioteer (higher mind) to grasp the reins (lower mind) and start giving direction to the horses. This training is called *sadhana*, the Sanskrit word for "spiritual practice." Through sadhana, we train all these aspects of ourselves so we ultimately experience the still, silent, eternal, and wise center called the Self, soul, or consciousness. Remember, it is from the vast, quiet space of consciousness, or our true Self, that we experience insight and the awakening of blocked energies. When everything is working in harmony, the Self makes the decisions and directs the body and mind with wisdom and love. The Sun Salutation practice you've been doing is an example of an introductory sadhana.

We all know how tempting it is to give in to our senses and how easy it is to become distracted, whether it's by scrolling on our phones, engaging in gossip, buying things we don't need, overeating, or staying in relationships that don't serve our higher purpose.

We've heard the popular saying "Follow your heart." The yogis would say: "Follow your purpose." Honor your feelings while being careful not to let your emotions and impulses distract you and carry you away from your svadharma. Our impulses come from our lower, conditioned mind. If we let ourselves eat junk food every time we crave it or react to anger with anger for decades, we will end up hurting ourselves even though, in the moment, acting on our emotions feels so good. Let your choices come from your higher mind, the one that takes time to distinguish between preya and shreya. When we are rooted in our motivation to experience shreya, we are driven by an intention to honor our potential and the welfare of others, and we direct our horses wisely.

This doesn't mean we become rigid workaholics and don't take time to enjoy a walk in the park with our children, an afternoon tea with a friend, or an entire day of self-care. We celebrate each moment with our motivation firm, knowing that all of it (vital rest and playtime included) is helping us realize our full human potential.

Samskaras

That critical movement of picking up the reins and guiding our horses differently, away from distractions and toward alignment with our deepest truths, requires an indomitable will. Every time we choose shreya over preya — even if it is a small act, such as reaching for a handful of almonds instead of cookies or going for a twenty-minute walk instead of engaging in twenty minutes of scrolling — we strengthen our will.

Some of the most exhilarating moments in spiritual development are when we catch a thought or impulse surfacing that will move us into a ditch (preya), and we redirect the mind and body toward that which is nourishing and beneficial in the long term (shreya). To strengthen our will, we must go against the grain of our conditioning. Conditioning means that the connection between thought and action has become automatic, immediate, and out of our control.

Training the mind to build willpower and make better choices is extremely hard at first...and then it becomes thrilling. With practice, you aren't at the mercy of your conditionings, or *samskaras*. Samskaras are impressions in the mind that come from patterns of thinking, speaking, and acting. Every time you use your will, you begin to create a new thought pattern and neural pathway, a new samskara. With repetition, the neural pathway or samskara becomes established. As you exercise your will, you become the driver who's consciously responding to and shaping your life instead of passively reacting to it.

In my younger years, I thought that freedom meant doing whatever I wanted. I was wrong. True freedom is not being a slave to your every impulse. Freedom is being able to pause and consciously choose to act in ways that honor and benefit you and others in the long term.

Intelligent Regret

When receiving teachings on preya and shreya, often people start beating themselves up about decisions they've made in the past that haven't been in their best interest. This is the perfect time to practice intelligent regret, the opposite of dysfunctional guilt. When practicing intelligent regret, we recognize what we could have done better in our past, and we learn from it without guilting or shaming ourselves. Channel any frustration you feel with yourself into a commitment to make better choices now.

Mirror Neurons

In the 1990s, a group of neuroscientists directed by Giacomo Rizzolatti in Italy discovered a group of neurons in the frontal lobe of the brain that are activated not only when we do something but also when we observe someone else doing that same thing. They called this group of neurons "mirror neurons." These neurons help explain why we smile when we see someone else smile, even if we don't know why that person is smiling. It's also part of why we start feeling sad when we're around someone who's depressed and pessimistic.

Mirror neurons cause "emotional contagion." They are a part of our nervous system that influence us to mirror the words, thoughts, behaviors, character, and habits of those we spend time with. If our friends eat well, spend time in nature, and exercise regularly, we are more likely to adopt healthy lifestyle habits. Conversely, if they lead sedentary lives indoors, we may be less inclined to exercise and enjoy nature.

On many levels, we have choices of who and what we allow into our lives. As we change our choices, everything in our lives begins to shift.

You could not remove a single grain of sand from its place without thereby changing something throughout all parts of the immeasurable whole.

JOHANN GOTTLIEB FICHTE

Protect Your Energy, Overcome Distractions

You are sacred land. Choose your travelers wisely.

DELLA HICKS-WILSON

To set ourselves up to make better decisions, it's crucial to protect our energy — to be careful of who and what we allow into our lives.

The Katha Upanishad teaches us to protect our eleven gates: the two eyes, two nostrils, two ears, mouth, sexual organs, organs of elimination, navel, and crown of the head.

See your body as a temple. Just as you are careful about what you let into a sacred space, keeping it clean and free of clutter, be diligent about what you allow into your mind and body, as it will absolutely affect your thoughts, health, practice, and life. Be extremely careful of who you spend time with and what you watch, read, listen to, and eat. Everything and everyone around you impacts you.

None of us is an island. We are connected and sensitive, influenced by the energies surrounding us. On a path to strengthen the mind and make better choices, it's vital to be in the company of those who encourage and inspire us.

The Guard Your Gates practice below helps us understand how much the outside world influences us. The relationship between cause and effect is real. If you eat a lot of sugar, you're almost certain to get cavities. If you're around motivated people, you will feel motivated.

Week Seven Practices

1. Guard Your Gates

Identify the things you've been letting into your mind or body that are distracting and/or harming you. This can be types of food or drink, TV shows, influencers on social media, websites, people, or activities. In our modern world, we may need to be especially careful to guard our gates from constant notifications on our devices, scrolling, overeating, binge-watching shows, and other common distractions. Without judging yourself or anyone else, make a list — it's OK if it's long — of all the harmful influences you've been letting into your mind and body. Then, pinpoint: What are your top ten?

As you make this list, inquire within: When your horses (senses and emotions) are driven by the lower mind, which is conditioned and automatic, where do they lead you? Remember to observe yourself from the spacious, nonjudgmental presence of witnessing consciousness. Instead of beating yourself up for letting x, y, and z into your life, rejoice that your awareness is evolving and you are actively taking the reins to make better choices.

Make a commitment to guard your gates from at least five of the things you listed for the next five weeks: for example, "I will only check email twice a day," "I will check social media once a day for ten minutes," "I will take all notifications off my phone," "I will refrain from gossiping with friends," and "I will cut out processed foods that leave me depleted."

Replace each of those five things (many of which are distractions from living your best life) with something that helps you. For example, you might commit to spending twenty minutes every morning doing your Sun Salutation and Savasana practices instead of engaging in twenty minutes of scrolling. You might decide to play a game or read with your child or partner every night for twenty minutes instead of feeling disconnected from them. Lifting weights three times a week could replace you spending time feeling bad about being out of shape. Having a club soda every evening instead of alcohol or turning all devices off earlier in the night and getting more sleep could be great choices to improve your well-being.

Write down these five commitments in your notebook, along with today's date and the date you will complete this program five weeks from now. How does it feel to take hold of the reins and use your higher, discerning mind to protect your energy and shape your life? Does it feel like repression or transformation?

2. *Visualization to Support Guard Your Gates Practice*

To review, samskaras are impressions in the mind that come from patterns of thinking, speaking, and acting. As we engage in the practices I described above, we change harmful samskaras and create beneficial ones. We have already been doing this for several weeks now. For example, we identified the labels that limit us, burned them in a fire puja, and replaced them with the space of pure potentiality. Then, we acknowledged thoughts of self-doubt and replaced them with empowering thoughts using the Sun Salutation mantras.

This week, we begin to protect our energy from some of the things that deplete us and distract us from self-realization. When we begin to replace an old pattern with a new one, however, the enticement of the old pattern often remains strong. Let's take the example of replacing twenty minutes of scrolling upon waking up in the morning with your twenty-minute Sun Salutation and Savasana practice. Say you have been in the habit of looking at your phone first thing when you wake up for ten years. That groove in the mind is deep.

As you practice releasing the old samskara and create a new one, it is powerful to visualize the new pattern. Try it this week. For example, if you fail one morning to do your Sun Salutations and instead pick up your phone, forgive yourself. That night while you are in bed, visualize yourself getting up the next morning and enjoying your Sun Salutations. See yourself experiencing the new pattern. Relish the vision — the movement beautifully harmonized with the breath, the feeling of the body growing stronger and more open, and the inner quiet that is becoming a precious sanctuary. Give that vision energy, more energy than the old pattern. This will prepare you for success in the morning. Remember your new story: I CAN.

In the morning, if your hand goes to pick up the phone, pause, breathe, and again visualize yourself practicing Sun Salutations. Then, step in that direction. Go to the bathroom, change your clothes, get hydrated, walk into your practice space. Do this again and again, morning after morning, until there is a morning — and it will happen — when you don't even think of checking your phone when you wake up. Your hand won't move toward the phone at all. Instead, upon waking up, your feet will come to the ground, and you'll take the steps to prepare for your sadhana. The new groove is established.

3. Deepen Your Sun Salutation Practice

Continuing your daily Sun Salutation practice can be one of the five commitments you make this week. This includes taking a few minutes every day to read through the twelve Sun Salutation mantras to continue to familiarize yourself with them. It also includes practicing the twelve-step Sun Salutation movements with chakra awareness.

Remember, in appreciating and recognizing the twelve qualities of the sun, you open yourself to embodying them, creating a world of positivity and power within you. Through the Surya Namaskara practice, you also cultivate a sense of connection with the primary energy source. As you practice, your mind and body become charged with vitality and radiance, like the sun.

Committing to this practice is a perfect opportunity to cultivate willpower, discipline, patience, and perseverance — some of the qualities of a spiritual warrior reviewed in Week Three. As you practice this sadhana daily, you are establishing new samskaras, impressions in the mind that turn into habits of thinking, speaking, and acting. You are creating new neural pathways, rewiring the brain to believe in yourself and act upon your growing self-worth, confidence, and vitality.

Adopt a minimum daily practice of at least six Sun Salutations. Feel free to extend this to nine or twelve daily Sun Salutations. If you miss one day that's OK. Practice your Sun Salutations at least six days a week. As always, in your journal this week, write about how this practice affects you. You can respond to the following inquiries as you continue to bring chakra awareness to your practice:

- As I connect with the heart chakra in Mountain Pose, how can I expand the ways I love and let myself be loved?
- As I open the throat chakra in the second, fifth, eighth, and eleventh poses, is there something inside of me that I wish to express? By whom would I like to be heard?
- As the lower belly activates in the third, seventh, and tenth poses, connecting me to my emotions and creative energy, what is stirred up within me?
- As the pineal gland (or third eye) is activated in the fourth and ninth poses, what do I see, imagine, and/or intuit?
- As the solar plexus chakra is engaged in the sixth pose, my belly and willpower strengthen. How does this feel?

As you become more familiar with the twelve mantras this week, inquire within:

- *Om Mitraya Namah:* How can I be a better friend to myself or another?
- *Om Ravaye Namah:* As I visualize taking in the radiance and light of the sun, does it inspire me to change in particular ways?
- *Om Suryaye Namah:* As I receive the sun's dynamic energy, what meaningful actions am I inspired to initiate?

Continue in this way with the remaining nine mantras. Review their meanings on pages 124–26 and write down your reflections.

Week Seven Daily Practice Sequence

In your daily journaling this week, include the five harmful samskaras you are working to replace and the beneficial ones you are cultivating in their place.

1. In My Own Hands: fifteen seconds
2. Optimal Breath practice: three minutes at the beginning of the day
3. All-Day Yoga
4. Review the meanings of the twelve Sun Salutation mantras: ten minutes
5. Sun Salutations with chakra awareness: fifteen minutes
6. Witness Meditation: six minutes
7. Savasana: five minutes
8. Journaling: five to ten minutes
9. Klesha Trigger Log: five to ten minutes at the end of the day

Total daily practice time: approximately fifty to sixty minutes

Week Seven Mitra Meeting

Let your mitras know how you have chosen to guard your gates through the duration of this program. What are the five new habits you are replacing your old distractions with? Pledge to be one another's accountability partners. Promise one another that you will call or text if and when you slip up. Cultivating new habits is hard. Celebrate your efforts with your mitras.

This week, you might want to share about how your breath practice, Witness Meditation, and Klesha Trigger Log are going. Also, how did your Sun Salutation practice feel this week? What are you learning from the chakra awareness and from getting familiar with the twelve mantras?

Key Terms from Week Seven

Preya: Pleasant in the moment, can be harmful in the long term.

Shreya: Difficult in the moment, beneficial in the long term.

Eleven gates: The two eyes, two nostrils, two ears, mouth, sexual organs, organs of elimination, navel, and crown of the head.

Samskara: Impressions in the mind that come from patterns of thinking, speaking, and acting.

Sadhana: Spiritual practice.

Tat Tvam Asi: "You are that"; in other words, you are the one who can transform your mind, health, and reality.

THE SUMMIT OF WISDOM

Be Established in Who You Truly Are

"Those who live in wisdom, how do they talk,
walk, sit, and move through this world?"
"They see themselves in all beings,
and all beings in themselves."

BHAGAVAD GITA (2.54–56)

I am another you.

MAYAN TEACHING

Yoga is rooted in a perennial philosophy that points to an ultimate truth introduced in Week Four: There is a changeless reality that underlies the world of change, and it is the essence of all beings. The purpose of spiritual practice is to experience this reality directly. Although it defies expression, ultimate reality is often described as all-pervading love, immeasurable possibility, and infinite light. Through spiritual disciplines such as yoga, we pursue direct experience of this truth and become radiant physically, mentally, and spiritually.

The Upanishads implore us to see the essence of all beings. The Mundaka Upanishad (600 BCE) expresses:

Deep in the heart of every creature dwells the seed of Love.
See the love in all.
Serve the love in all.
Be at peace, attaining the summit of wisdom. (2.5–6)

The Amritabindu Upanishad conveys: *I have realized the Self
who is present in all beings. I am united with Love.* According to the
Paramahansa Upanishad, *the illumined ones serve love and live for
the welfare of all. United with love, serene, a source of joy and wisdom, they rest in love, are supported by the staff of wisdom, and reside
in the Unitive state.*

To know that the essence of all beings is the same and to live
in accord with this awareness is to be in the unitive state of yoga.
When we realize our fundamental unity, the tendencies toward hatred, separation, preferences, and aversion diminish. We recognize
that all beings possess an equal right to life, fostering empathy and
compassion. We become incapable of ignoring injustices inflicted
upon any individual, animal, or the planet.

The Chandogya Upanishad describes a secret dwelling place in
the lotus of the heart. It is a love that knows we are all connected and
made of the same divine light. Union with this secret dwelling place
births a peaceful and purposeful state. To intimately experience the
love and radiance that is the essence of our being, we peel away the
layers that block it.

*Your task is not to seek for love, but merely to seek and find
all the barriers within yourself that you have built against it.*

RUMI

In Week One, we began to open up to our mitras, and some of
those layers fell away. In Week Two, we acknowledged our kleshas,
and more layers peeled off. In Week Three, we became aware of the

subtle body — the world of thoughts and emotions and how they shape our physical reality. With this awareness of the subtle body, we began to link breath with movement. Blocks began to loosen in the energetic and the physical body. In Week Four, we met ourselves — the pleasant, the painful, and everything in between — from the open, welcoming, nonjudgmental presence of the witness. A few more layers softened. In the fire puja we performed in Week Five, we shed more layers. As we changed limiting thoughts in Week Six and chose shreya over preya in Week Seven, even more layers came off. Each time we replace a harmful samskara with a nurturing one, layers fall away.

Congratulations on the work you have done so far. Rejoice in your efforts. You are becoming a spiritual warrior. We will keep doing these practices again and again. Patience and repetition are essential on this path. Remember, results can seem slow to come, but we are practicing to cultivate lasting inner peace, radiant health, and a foundation upon which to live to our greatest capacity. Be happy for the seeds you are planting.

This week, we will peel away more layers to prepare ourselves to ultimately yoke with our essence. Our surface-level personalities shift and change as we go through different phases of our lives. For a few years, we may try one profession, and then we move to another. For some years, we may feel antagonistic toward a certain person or group of people. Then, one day, we come to an understanding and perhaps forgiveness. For weeks, we may be reclusive, wanting only to spend time with ourselves. Quiet evenings reading a book are a treasure. Then we feel like being social, enjoying dinners and gatherings with friends and community. On many levels, we are beings who change all the time.

Though our personality and activities may shift, that which lies at the core of our being is unchanging. If we can keep our awareness on the love that is always present within us, we can connect with each other with much more ease, even if our interests, personalities, races, religions, ethnicities, genders, or nationalities are different. More layers release.

In the Yoga Sutras, Patanjali describes avidya as the klesha that is at the root of all other kleshas. *Vidya* means "wisdom." The prefix *a-* means "not." *Avidya* literally means "not wisdom." It is commonly translated as "confusion or delusion" — mistaking illusion for reality. It refers to ignorance of the true Self as being interconnected with all life and made of the same essence. Kleshas such as anger, hate, and jealousy can stem from losing sight of the fact that we all share a common ground.

The opposite of avidya is wisdom. In this context, wisdom is knowing that, in our essence, we are not similar to one another — we are identical. The same light moves through all of us, though it is expressed in our distinct ways. Underlying all our surface differences, we are united by a shared foundation. We all want peace, security, safety, and freedom from pain. We all want to love and be loved. We are all born and our bodies will die. Being aware of our shared essence opens our heart to empathize with another's sorrows instead of being indifferent, to rejoice in another's accomplishments instead of feeling jealous, and to feel compassion for another's pain.

As cited in the beginning of this chapter, in the Bhagavad Gita, Arjuna asks Krishna, "Those who live in wisdom, how do they talk, walk, sit, and move through this world?" Krishna responds, "They see themselves in all beings, and all beings in themselves" (2.54–56). The Sanskrit greeting *Namaste* means: "I bow to the light that connects us and reminds us that we are fundamentally the same." Imagine beginning every encounter with this sentiment. Could the use and understanding of this greeting help us avoid creating or deepening the wounds of division?

The legacy that yoga gives humanity is to ultimately see one another as kin. *Vasudhaiva Kutumbakam* — "The world is one family" in Sanskrit — was my grandfather's favorite Vedic teaching. He was a yogi as well as a freedom fighter alongside Mahatma Gandhi during India's struggle for independence from British colonialism in the 1940s. He experienced the horrors of war and the bloodshed that took place, not only between the British and Indians but also between Hindus and Muslims as the country was divided into India and Pakistan.

In 2015, I went to Khaknar, a tribal village in Madhya Pradesh, central North India, where my grandfather lived. At ninety-four years old, he was nearing the end of his life. My grandfather, whom I called Bapuji, had been healthy and vibrant most of his life. Since his teenage years, he had maintained a daily morning yoga practice, including asana, pranayama, meditation, and contemplation inspired by the ancient texts. He often said that his morning practice provided him with the energy he needed to serve others throughout the day.

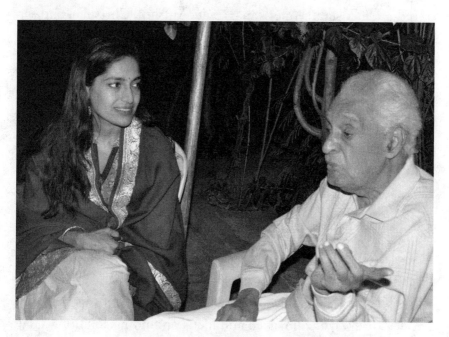

FIGURE 11: Bapuji and I in Khaknar in 2015.

Bapuji's career spanned education and international development. While living in New Delhi, he helped bring educational radio and TV to India and then moved to Maryland to work for the Washington County Board of Education. He then spent several years living in various countries while serving UNESCO. The final three decades of his life were devoted to rural development in Khaknar. There, he raised funds to build the village's first hospital, primary and secondary schools, and a vocational training center. He also established a community center, offering workshops in women's literacy, participation in village governments, modern farming techniques, and yoga. Additionally, he created a stage for children to perform music, dance, and theater. I saw many bright and happy faces of children in that space.

Knowing this was the last time I would see him, I asked, "Bapuji, if there was one piece of wisdom you could give to the next generation, what would it be?" His response was: "Forget these labels of Indian, Pakistani, American, Hindu, Muslim, Christian, and see each other as human. Universal brotherhood and sisterhood are the foundations of love."

Bapuji's words offer a profound lesson in yoga and a pathway to peace. In a world increasingly marked by division, I find myself returning to these words often. When my own thoughts veer toward divisiveness — whether in matters of politics, health, or social issues — I try to catch myself and redirect my mind toward connection and understanding.

For example, in discussions around yoga and cultural appropriation, it's undeniable that the essence of yoga is sometimes lost in modern settings. The way yoga has been adapted in the West often disconnects it from its spiritual roots. While this can be painful to witness, compassion is always an option. We can come together with respect for everyone involved and focus on finding solutions. How can we deepen our understanding of yoga and better represent it?

How can we improve yoga teacher training programs? How can we distill the most potent wisdom and practices of a deep tradition and bring them into the modern world in relevant and impactful ways?

This book is a part of that effort, helping practitioners and teachers better understand and represent yoga. We can engage in this important work without spending energy on blame or shame, which perpetuates pain and division. Instead of creating or furthering separation, we can seize the opportunity to collaborate and enjoy the process of learning and growing as a collective.*

Bapuji's teachings and life experiences remind me that whenever our mind creates a sense of separation between ourselves and others, we have a choice: to listen to diverse viewpoints, seek understanding, and find solutions, or to succumb to judgment and division, which often leads to hostility and alienation. Each of us has the power to guide our minds in a direction that fosters connection rather than separation.

Figure 12 shows the cover of my grandfather's 1990 book *Towards Global Consciousness*. The same mandala image graces the entrance of the community center he established in Khaknar, called Manav Mandir, or "Temple of Humanity."

Wisdom Is Wisdom

In 2003, I had the opportunity to spend three weeks in a small Brazilian village in the state of Acre, located in the Amazonian rainforest bordering Peru. In the Amazon, I learned that wisdom is wisdom. We can get attached to labels like "Hindu," "Indian," "yoga," "shamanism" — *this* tradition, *that* country. The ego grasps at these identities,

---

* I offer additional insights on a unitive perspective on yoga and cultural appropriation, including a story about Khaknar, in an article I wrote for *Elephant Journal*. Visit https://www.elephantjournal.com/2021/11/yoga-cultural -appropriation-why-we-can-heal-the-world-with-kindness-reema-datta.

creating a story, a sense of belonging. This can be comforting on one level, but on another, it can create separation between self and others. The more we cling to the labels and identities that we or society apply to ourselves, the more we can forget that even though we may be different on the surface, we are the same in our essence.

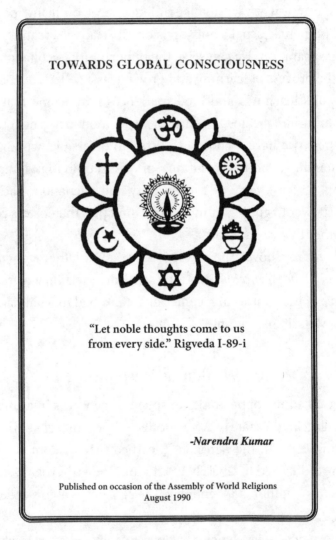

TOWARDS GLOBAL CONSCIOUSNESS

"Let noble thoughts come to us
from every side." Rigveda I-89-i

-Narendra Kumar

Published on occasion of the Assembly of World Religions
August 1990

FIGURE 12: The cover of my grandfather's book
Towards Global Consciousness (1990). The same mandala graces
the entrance of his community center.

In Brazil, we engaged in a light diet and sometimes fasted. Fasting is a common ritual among yogis in India, as is eating light, balanced meals. In the Amazon, we danced in a circle — rhythmic, steady movement that helped to settle the mind. This reminded me of the rhythmic flow of asana as well as of *garba*, folk dances of India that I grew up participating in. The shamans sang gentle, soothing songs to us. The way the songs relaxed and opened my body and mind reminded me of the mantras I grew up hearing my mom and grandmothers sing.

Eventually, after all the ritual — the fasting, movement, songs, and interaction with community — we sat under the stars of the vast Amazonian sky immersed in our own quietude. It was just like yoga, where we use a light, nourishing diet, movement, and song as preliminary practices to help settle the mind and body so we can eventually sit still and meditate.

"Stay connected to your breath," the woman shaman said to me as the communal ceremony came to an end and the personal inner journey became the focus. *How similar to yoga*, I thought to myself. Whatever happens, the most important part of any yoga practice is to stay connected to the breath, which is our bridge from the outer world to the inner.

In the jungle, I experienced Spirit as an unconditionally loving energy. The more I stayed with my breath, the more I felt this all-embracing, forgiving, deeply nourishing energy everywhere. The line between inner and outer dissolved. As I felt Spirit's power, I felt my own. I felt secure and protected, indestructible and free. There was no separation — no line where I ended and Spirit began. We were one being. Seamless.

Afterward, I realized that what I'd experienced in the Amazon was what a yogi would call yoga: union. A central teaching of yoga is that separation is an illusion. We're all connected to each other and to Source. We all carry infinite light and potential. Realizing this wisdom directly and intimately, with every fiber of your being, is the antidote to the root klesha, avidya — mistaking the illusion of separation for reality.

I recount this story of my experience in the Amazon to emphasize that yoga's central message of oneness — our shared essence and interconnection with all life — is found in indigenous communities worldwide. Spiritual and shamanic traditions around the globe point to the interconnectedness of all life and have practices to help us experience and reexperience the oneness of life so we can live with an awareness of our unity and potential.

Foundational to both Indian and Tibetan medicine is the understanding that ignorance of the interconnectedness of life is the primary cause of disease, because it leads us to feel alone, unsupported, anxious, and stressed. If we think we are different and separate, we can feel weak, lost, and lonely and not have the strength or motivation to get up and offer the gifts we were born to contribute. Knowing our true state of unity gives us strength, courage, motivation, and purpose.

The teachings of oneness emphasized in wisdom traditions across the globe are also recognized by many in Western science. For example, Einstein's work reflects the idea that we are all interconnected within a vast energy field. Quantum physicists agree that all of life is interconnected and our energies affect one another and the whole of existence.

The ancient yogis urge us to be aware of our common ground and to recognize that *the separation we create in our minds between self and other leads to the division and violence prevalent in the world.* As vastly different as our histories, backgrounds, and life experiences are, we share a fundamental unity. This is not to deny our diverse cultures and backgrounds. We can celebrate and honor our diversity while also transcending it, always aware of the unity that underlies our existence.

Many spiritual traditions and indigenous communities world-wide also hold that the Divine lives inside each being. The lyrics of a traditional South American *icaro* (a Quechua word for a medicine song) say, "The medicine that cures me is the medicine that cures everyone: We are all God." The Gita conveys a similar message, teaching us to "see the Self" in all beings (5.7). "The Self" refers to the soul, which is inseparable from the Divine.

In sum, yoga practices and philosophy have the following in common with spiritual traditions across the world:

- Motivation to heal oneself for the benefit of the collective
- The asking of blessings from guardians
- Fasting or a light diet
- Singing
- Breath awareness
- Rhythmic movement
- Meditation
- Direct experience and reexperience of eternal and liberating truths such as the unity underlying all phenomena

Yoga emphasizes daily practice because we want an experience of connection and unity to be our natural state, not an extraordinary, miraculous achievement. *The Yogi's Way* dives deep into working through kleshas, because we won't be able to maintain unity consciousness for long when the mind is cluttered and overcome with disturbances.

This ancient wisdom has been passed down from teacher to student as an unbroken tradition for thousands of years. In the last few decades, many behavioral scientists are beginning to uncover the healing value of love and connection. Research studies provide empirical evidence of the effects of love and positive social connections across various domains of health. For example, a study found that individuals in satisfying marriages exhibit lower levels of stress hormones, reduced inflammation, and stronger immune function compared to those in less satisfying marriages. The findings of a 2010 study suggest that social isolation can lead to higher blood pressure. In a comprehensive review, the psychologist and researcher Sheldon Cohen discussed the evidence linking social relationships to various health outcomes, including mortality, cardiovascular health, immune function, and mental well-being. He emphasized the importance of fostering positive social connections for health promotion as well as disease prevention.

Eternal Truth

As mentioned in the introduction, the teachings in this book draw from the original texts of yogic wisdom, including the Vedas, Upanishads, Bhagavad Gita, and Yoga Sutras. Vedic sages called the enduring and universal principles within these texts Sanatana Dharma, meaning "Eternal Truth." These teachings came to the first yogis while they were in states of deep meditation. Anyone who goes into a receptive meditative state will experience similar realizations. This is why the core teachings of these texts are found in spiritual and shamanic traditions throughout the world. Many scientific studies are beginning to provide evidence of some of these truths, which have such common themes as the power of the mind to affect our physical health, our interconnection with all life, and the "pure potentiality" that physicists describe as the underlying reality of all phenomena. We all carry these truths in our essence.

In the Bhagavad Gita, Krishna says, "All paths lead to Me" (4.11). "Me" can be understood as Christ Consciousness, Krishna Consciousness, or the consciousness of any being from any tradition who has realized the eternal truth of unity. Many of Christ's teachings, such as loving your neighbor and seeing yourself as the light of the world, are similar to Vedic principles.

Approximately *five thousand* years after Sanatana Dharma was established, it became known as Hinduism, a term coined in the nineteenth century during British colonial rule. The word *Hindu* originates from the Persian term for people living around the Indus River. It referred to people from a specific region, rather than a particular religion.

Rooted in Sanatana Dharma, Hinduism embraces the belief that all religions are branches of the same mighty tree. Truth has always been universal, but the same truth can be viewed from many standpoints. As my grandfather used to explain, "When water is poured into vessels of different shapes, it takes the shape of the vessel, but the water itself is the same."

According to Hindu philosophy, every human being and every religion has an individuality worthy of reverence. This path recognizes that the quest for truth is personal — whether one finds it in God, multiple deities, or intellectual pursuits.

While growing up in the United States, I remember feeling uncomfortable when non-Indian friends or adults asked me what religion I was. "Hindu," I would say, feeling my face flush. I could sense I was being judged and misunderstood as someone who was part of a strange culture of idol worshippers. When my sixth-grade social studies teacher in Maryland asked me this question, upon hearing the response of my twelve-year-old self, she said in a surprised and condescending tone, "Oh, I thought your family was more modern than that."

I understand that Hinduism can be confusing. Rather than a rigid set of dogmas, it is a way of life rich with yogic wisdom and practices that nurture our potential and foster a direct experience of eternal truths. All the gods and goddesses in the Hindu pantheon represent aspects of ourselves. For example, Durga represents our courage. Saraswati symbolizes the creativity and knowledge that live within us. Rama represents our capacity for inner peace even when life gets extremely difficult. Shiva reflects our ability to let go of what no longer serves us to create space for new possibilities.

Yoga is meant to awaken each of us to our potential. When we gaze upon or sing to a deity, we revive the qualities within ourselves that the deity represents. Everything is within us. Yet we forget. We get disconnected from our capacity. We get distracted by external influences that tell us we need so many things outside of ourselves to be whole and happy. Our rituals, ceremonies, and festivals are moments when we come together to rekindle the many facets of the light we were born with and that live within us. We do all this to feed the story "I AM that infinite and immutable spirit who is worthy and capable of being brave, wise, loving, and creative. I CAN share my gifts fully and realize my potential."

Heaven and hell are within us. All the Gods and Goddesses and all the worlds are within us. This is the great realization of the Upanishads of India in the 9th Century BC.

HUSTON SMITH

Cutting-edge neuroscientists, physicists, and medical practitioners are echoing the wisdom not only of my elders and ancestors but of wisdom keepers worldwide. Medical professionals now prescribe chanting Om, backed by research demonstrating how its three sounds — *a*, *u*, and *m* — stimulate the vagus nerve, inducing the body's natural relaxation response and fostering a sense of interconnection. Doctors, therapists, educators, coaches, and healthcare professionals increasingly recommend pranayama, asana, mantra, and meditation to their clients. To fully benefit from these practices, it's crucial to recognize the philosophy that underlies them. Practicing with wisdom and understanding unlocks more profound transformations.

Week Eight Practices

1. Contemplate the Klesha of Delusion

To summarize, the Yoga Sutras identify the root klesha as avidya, which means "without wisdom." This refers to a basic ignorance of who we truly are and of the underlying reality that connects everything in the Universe. Yoga philosophy emphasizes that the same limitless light and potential live within each of us as our true Self. This light unifies us and helps us to see one another as kin who belong to one global family. It can help reduce our experience of other kleshas, such as anger, hatred, and jealousy. This not only opens us to the healing force of love that lives inside us but plants seeds for a more peaceful world.

We may not even be aware of the anger, fear, and separation we carry in the depths of our minds. The teachings of this tradition ask us to go deep into the recesses of our mind, practice a radical humility, and find the divisiveness we carry within. Remember, yogis welcome a questioning mind. Let your practice be the ground for your own realizations. Take some time to contemplate the following questions in the quietness of your own heart:

- Have I sacrificed the welfare of any person, animal, or the planet for my own profit, pleasure, or prestige (such as a higher salary, a better home, a more comfortable life)?
- Do I carry assumptions about people who come from a different background than me? What are they?
- Do I care for my neighbors and fellow humans as I do for my own family and friends? Or do I perceive and act with a sense of separation, indifference, or aversion toward them?
- How does it feel to see myself as a separate being, living on my own island, versus as a wave in an ocean, connected to Source and all beings?

- How does it feel to honor the labels I identify with while being deeply rooted in humanity's fundamental unity? Any shifts in the mind or heart to note?
- In what moments does my mind become divisive? How can I redirect it toward understanding and connection?
- Have I internalized scripts that block me from love in my personal life? That prevent me from experiencing connection?

We all share the wound of fragmentation
and we can all share in the cure of unification.

GABRIELLE ROTH

2. Savor a Joy Date

Another eternal truth is that joy is our birthright. In many stories of deities such as Radha, Krishna, Sita, and Ram, they delight in nature, beauty, art, and music while taking care of their worldly responsibilities. Once a week for the next five weeks, take time to do something that gives you pure joy. Let there be no reason other than that you love it. It can be something different each week. Perhaps one week it is sitting outside watching the sunset and listening to the world quiet down. Perhaps another week it is taking a walk and sitting under a tree to read a book. Another week, it could be meeting up with a friend whom you haven't seen for ages. Maybe another week it is playing your favorite songs and dancing your heart out in your living room.

Whatever it is, do it, not because the physical exercise is good for you or because the social contact is healthy, but only because it makes your heart happy. As you choose your weekly joy date, feel boundless in your mind and free of judgment. What will you do this week?

3. Deepen Your Sun Salutation Practice

Practice six to twelve Sun Salutations daily this week. If you feel comfortable, you may begin to incorporate mantra into your practice. One approach is to say one mantra at the beginning of each Sun Salutation. If the Sanskrit feels challenging right now, use the English translation. Either way, remember the meaning and significance of the mantra. Then, do the set of twelve poses with chakra awareness.

For example, the first three rounds of Sun Salutations might look like this:

1. Starting in Mountain Pose, say, "Om Mitraya Namah" and/ or "The universal friend who is friendly and affectionate to oneself and others." Remember, as you say this out loud, in a whisper, or silently, you plant seeds in your mind to embody this quality of the sun. Connect with your heart chakra and move through the twelve poses with chakra awareness. Integrate the mantra's meaning throughout the sequence.

2. Again in Mountain Pose, say, "Om Ravaye Namah" and/or "The bestower of radiance and light that inspires change." Practice the twelve poses with chakra awareness. Internalize the mantra's meaning as you move through the sequence.

3. Back once more in Mountain Pose, say, "Om Suryaye Namah" and/or "The dispeller of darkness who induces action." Practice the twelve poses with chakra awareness. Embed the mantra's meaning into the movement.

On day 1 of this week, continue like this for three more Sun Salutations so that you practice at least six Sun Salutations with the first six mantras and with chakra awareness. The next day, do the same thing with the next six mantras. Alternate like this throughout the week.

To see a visual of this practice and follow it online, visit The YogisWay.com/thebook.

4. Refresh Your Journaling

This week, as a part of your journaling practice, reflect on the following questions:

- How is your six-minute Witness Meditation practice going (page 85)? How does it feel to be the witness of your thoughts, emotions, sensations, and experiences?
- How is the Klesha Trigger Log looking (page 42)? What are you noticing about what triggers your kleshas? Is this practice helping you build self-awareness and slow down your reactions?
- Consider the five new samskaras you began creating last week (page 148). How are you doing with those this week? How does it feel to guard your gates and protect your energy?
- What did you do for your joy date this week? How did it feel? What did it bring up for you?

Week Eight Daily Practice Sequence

1. In My Own Hands: fifteen seconds
2. Optimal Breath practice: three minutes at the beginning of the day
3. All-Day Yoga
4. Sun Salutations with chakra awareness and mantras: fifteen to twenty minutes
5. Witness Meditation: six minutes

6. Savasana: five minutes
7. Journaling: five to ten minutes
8. Klesha Trigger Log: five to ten minutes at the end of the day

Total daily practice time: approximately forty to fifty-five minutes

Week Eight Mitra Meeting

Discuss your reflections from this chapter with your mitras. What do the teachings on avidya bring up for you? As you become more familiar with the practices you've learned so far, go deeper with yourself and your mitras. Practice honesty and courage. Keep the inner gaze curious with a goal of understanding rather than judging. What are you learning about yourself? What are you struggling with? How do these practices feel in your mind, body, and spirit? What questions and insights are arising? Talk these through with your mitras.

Key Terms from Week Eight

Vidya: Wisdom.

Avidya: Not wisdom, which leads to delusion and confusion.

Vasudhaiva Kutumbakam: "The world is one family."

Sanatana Dharma: The timeless and universal principles that form the foundation of Vedic wisdom, including yoga; translates as "Eternal Truth."

ALCHEMY

Check Your Heart, Change Your Thoughts

*Since you alone are responsible for your thoughts,
only you can change them.*

Paramahansa Yogananda

Think globally, act locally.

Anonymous

Through yoga, we loosen granthis — knots in the subtle body — which keep us from experiencing our full potential, our true Self. As long as we are hurting ourselves or others, we can't be authentic or grow on our spiritual path. When we say, do, or think something harmful about ourselves or someone else, we affect the pranic winds in the subtle body, creating or deepening blocks within, and our mind won't be free to expand into its full capacity.

In this chapter, you will learn an awareness practice to help you notice your thoughts, words, actions, and choices in ten fundamental ways. This practice supports you in choosing thoughts, words, and actions that don't hurt you or others but foster fulfillment, peace, and freedom.

Awareness: If This, Then That

Today we have a lot of options when it comes to how to live. It's our responsibility to make choices that lead to harmony rather than pain for ourselves, others, and the planet. Spiritual traditions across the globe teach us to take responsibility for what we experience, because our thoughts, words, and actions affect our personal reality. The first step in this process is awareness.

The Bible teaches, "As ye sow, so shall ye reap" (Galatians 6:7). Saint Francis of Assisi beautifully expressed this further: "It is in giving that we receive." The yogis teach *karma*: Our actions, words, and thoughts have consequences. All these wisdom traditions have this very important principle in common. The choices we make in each moment plant seeds for our future experiences.

As we've discussed in these pages, according to quantum physicists, the world is a field of pure potentiality. We experience life on the basis of the impressions in our minds. We can't necessarily control the outside world, but we can choose the way we respond to it and the impressions that our own thoughts, words, and actions make on our mind.

For example, we can choose to live in a world where we help our neighbors even if we don't know their names, or we can live in a world where all we see is separation. Spirituality is about changing ourselves in order to change the world. Everything starts with our own thoughts.

With the help of his mitra, Arjuna placed all his energy on working through the chaos within his own mind. Only after delving deep into inner reflection to clear and ground his mind did he take steps to lead his people out of an oppressive regime in which the rulers were fueled by greed, selfishness, and deception. Arjuna's story is still relevant, as many of us aspire to reshape a world marred by injustice and cruelty. When we acknowledge and heal our own wounds, we prepare ourselves to confront the tragedy of injustice with understanding and empathy for all those involved. This is far from easy, but we are building a foundation within to do so.

Act for justice, but be driven by love, else this will never end.

Dr. Lisette Garcia

Presence

It takes a great amount of awareness to be present and cognizant of our thoughts, words, and actions in each moment. It is only in the now, when we are truly present, that we can consciously create different experiences in our life. However, we have become a culture of multitasking in which we make decisions in haste, do things quickly, and react without considering the consequences of our actions.

A reaction happens quickly when we are not in control of our mind. This often leads to words or behavior that we regret. As we cultivate an open and more relaxed mind, we can breathe, pause, and choose our responses wisely. This is not suppression. It is transformation. It is living in freedom and consciously planting seeds, with wisdom. When we respond from our intelligent, discerning higher mind, it is much more likely that our response will help the situation and the people involved rather than hurting ourselves and others and making things worse.*

Wisdom in Action

To be able to choose shreya over preya, we must cultivate healthy thinking habits. This week, we will continue to replace harmful thoughts with beneficial ones. The awareness practice outlined below

---

* In some circumstances, unthinking, quick action is appropriate and can prevent harm. For example, if you place your hand on a hot stove and reflexively pull it away, you will save yourself from a severe burn. In most circumstances, however, reacting without thinking leads to harm.

is influenced by the first two limbs of the eight-limbed path of yoga from the Yoga Sutras of Patanjali (circa 200 BCE).

Drawing from the *yamas* and *niyamas*, or moral disciplines and observances, we will develop awareness of our current patterns and cultivate habits that generate peace and well-being for ourselves, family, community, and the world.

The earliest mention of the yamas and niyamas is found in the Rigveda, the oldest known Vedic text, which was likely compiled around 1500 BCE. Teachings such as the Ten Commandments of Judaism and Christianity, the Ten Virtues of Buddhism, and *ho'opo-nopono*, a traditional Hawaiian practice, echo the message of the yamas and niyamas. All these practices help us refine our thoughts, words, and actions to live a simple, compassionate, and clean life in which we don't create pain for ourselves or anyone else. There are many teachings across wisdom traditions throughout the world that express similar principles. After all, wisdom is wisdom.

Purify yourself by a well-ordered and useful life. Watch over your thoughts, feelings, words, and actions. This will clear your vision.

Sri Nisargadatta Maharaj

Yamas

Yamas are ethical principles that are difficult and yet vitally important to apply to daily life. These principles are universal. Whatever your background, you can use the five main yamas as a guide to cultivate self-awareness and ethical behavior.

The Five Main Yamas

- *Ahimsa:* Nonviolence, compassion. Avoid any cruel, destructive thoughts and comments about yourself and others. Be gentle in your thoughts, words, and actions.

- **Satya:** Truth. Be honest with yourself and others. Saying or doing anything from a place of truth and love is usually less painful than what avoidance or untruth brings in the long run.
- **Asteya:** Nonstealing. Honor people's property, time, talents, relationships, and resources. When one of these is offered, take only as much as you need, so you are not depriving someone else. Develop a sense of abundance, confidence, and self-reliance.
- **Brahmacharya:** Observe moderation in all things, nourish relationships, identify with the light that exists within all beings, honor commitments and boundaries, be responsible in sexual behavior.
- **Aparigraha:** Nongrasping; nonaccumulation; freedom from possessiveness, greed, and covetousness. Let go of what you don't need. Practice simple acts of generosity.

Niyamas

Niyamas are personal observances that focus on our relationship with our own mind, body, and environment. They bring us closer to consciousness — the deeper, connected part of ourselves that is inherently loving, wise, generous, and peaceful.

The Five Main Niyamas

- **Saucha:** Cleanliness. This relates to both your physical space (home, work) as well as your mind. Every object in your home or work environment takes up a space in your mind. Free yourself of what you don't need or use. This will help declutter the mind.
- **Santosha:** Contentment. Be grateful for what you have.

Release jealousy by rejoicing in what others have. Empathize with others' misfortunes.

- **Tapas:** Discipline, passion, burning zeal, fiery determination. Is your will strong today, or do you need to confide in a mitra for encouragement, listen to an inspiring story, attend a community event, spend time in nature, or anything else to reignite your zeal?

- **Svadhyaya:** Self-reflection, self-study. Observe yourself without judgment. What have you learned today about your strengths, weaknesses, passions, purpose, and destructive or nourishing habits? Do you keep the space of your heart and mind open and receptive?

- **Ishvara pranidhana:** Surrender, trust. Everything happens for a purpose. Receive the lessons. Allow doors to close and open.

The Practice of Developing Awareness:
Check Your Heart, Change Your Thoughts

Watch your thoughts; they become words. Watch your words;
they become actions. Watch your actions; they become habits.
Watch your habits; they become character.
Watch your character; for it becomes your destiny.

KATHA UPANISHAD (4.4.5)

Check Your Heart, Change Your Thoughts (CYH) is a highly structured journaling practice that offers a way for you to observe your choices and change your patterns around the ten yamas and niyamas each day. To do it, you look back to the previous forty-eight hours and consider these three items for each yama and niyama in turn:

- A plus sign (+), after which you write how well you did with that yama or niyama on that day (or the day before), and you celebrate it.
- A minus sign (−) to log instances when you didn't follow the principle so well.
- Action items: notes on how you can respond better next time.

When I first learned this practice, I thought, *I am the most horrible person in the world!* Soon, I realized that everyone who engages in this awareness practice has the same response. When you begin this week's exercise, please remember: You are not a terrible person. You are someone who is growing in awareness, love, and compassion. This exercise is another opportunity to practice intelligent regret instead of dysfunctional guilt. With intelligent regret, you learn from the past and understand how you can act differently now. Instead of shaming yourself, rejoice in the fact that your awareness is expanding. As you practice daily, your awareness will become more refined. Ultimately, *your awareness will become your teacher and healer.* You will find yourself becoming a light to others and experiencing life with more joy and fulfillment.

Here is an example of what a completed CYH journal practice might look like.

---

1. **Ahimsa:** Nonviolence. Gentle and meaningful thoughts, words, actions.
   + Noticed my friend start to gossip. I changed the subject, so we wouldn't waste our energy in meaningless talk and judgment.
   − Spoke harshly to a family member and to myself.
   Action: Breathe deeply and pause before speaking,

especially when I know I'm being triggered. Notice the inner critic and befriend it while not giving in to it.

2. **Satya:** Be truthful all day to yourself and others.

   + Woke up feeling really down. Took a shower, put on nice clothes, looked in the mirror, and told myself that I am enough.

   – Tried to convince myself that I like my job, but I don't.

   Action: Spend ten quiet minutes in nature every day so that I can slowly get in touch with what I really want in my career. Shut off all devices and either sit under a tree or go for a walk by myself.

3. **Asteya:** Refrain from stealing. Honor other people's property, time, talents, and resources.

   + My best friend's three kids were sick. I really wanted to talk to her for advice. I practiced self-restraint and meditated instead.

   – Left a friend's house in a rush after my kid had a playdate there. I didn't have a chance to help clean up the mess the kids made.

   Action: On the weekend, coordinate a time with this friend to come to her house and help clean. If she says no, bring her and her family one of her favorite dishes.

4. **Brahmacharya:** Nourish relationships. See the light in all beings. Honor commitments. Engage in responsible sexual behavior.

   + I went out for dinner with coworkers. One of them, who is married, was sitting a little too close to me

and made a pass at me. I ended the conversation and
began to talk with someone else.

– Felt resentment toward a colleague when I saw her
post something divisive on social media.

Action: Remember that everyone is divine. Wish people who say and do hurtful things healing and understanding. Seek out opportunities to connect with
people who have different perspectives from mine.

5. **Aparigraha:** Nongrasping. Let go of what you don't need.
Practice generosity.

+ I cooked extra food for dinner. Instead of enjoying leftovers and not having to cook the next day, I gave the
extra food to my neighbor. She's an elderly woman
living alone and has no family in town.

– A coworker expressed that she needed help. I had the
time and energy to do it but made an excuse and
rushed home to watch my favorite show.

Action: Speak to this colleague tomorrow and tell her I'd
be happy to help after hours.

6. **Saucha:** Cleanliness. Keep the space in your home and
heart simple and clean.

+ I mopped the floors and washed the sheets and towels,
even though I was tempted to skip the chores for yet
another day.

– I let myself feel hurt by my partner's lack of communication. Instead of picking up the phone and clearing
the air, I've been avoidant. My mind feels clouded,
and my heart is heavy.

Action: Find the courage to be vulnerable and make the
phone call.

7. **Santosha:** Contentment. Rejoice in other people's successes. Be happy and grateful for what you have.

    + I felt happy that my sister bought land to build her dream house.

    − I felt jealous of a coworker who received a promotion at work.

    Action: Rejoice for my coworker and be grateful to know it's possible to be promoted. Create an action plan for what I need to do to be promoted and follow through with it.

8. **Tapas:** Fiery determination to live your purpose.

    + I made five phone calls today asking for much-needed help to move forward on a project close to my heart.

    − The voice of doubt paid a visit this morning and has been lingering all day.

    Action: Find someone who has the same problem as me and try to encourage them.

9. **Svadhyaya:** Self-reflection, self-study with the purpose to understand rather than judge.

    + When negative thoughts about myself arose today, I caught myself and played an uplifting song that I love. I danced for the length of the song.

    − A harmful phrase began to loop in my mind that I never have enough time, money, or friends. It went on for a long time.

    Action: Every night before I go to sleep, give thanks for what I have.

10. **Ishvara pranidhana:** Surrender and trust. Do you allow life to happen as it does, or do you resist what is?

+ I felt OK about having to find another place to live.

− I felt major resistance and anger about violence in my
   community.

Action: Catch the energy of the anger and use it as fuel
   to collaborate with neighbors on solutions.

Check Your Heart, Change Your Thoughts is not about judging yourself, another, or a situation in your life. It is about recognizing the choices we have in responding to the present moment. We must realize that our power comes from our thoughts, which fuel our words and actions. We can't control what happens to us. Our ability to heal and create a new reality lies in how we choose to respond to our current circumstances. Through our responses, we plant seeds for our future experiences, and in this way we shift our reality. Whatever we choose to think, say, and do shapes our personal reality. We get to choose what we think, say, and do in each moment.

Whether someone is laughing at me, screaming at me, or making a scene, I have a choice to react in a similar way — or I can pause, breathe, and respond with awareness. If I scream or make fun of someone, I plant the seeds to experience this kind of painful scenario again and again. If I breathe, send the person a silent wish to heal and be happy, and then go on with my day, I plant the seeds for a future of understanding and care. How do you want to respond in each moment, and what kind of future do you want to create?

We can judge a person or a situation, or we can make a commitment to change ourselves — because we can control ourselves. We can watch our mind. How does judging others and the world make you feel versus committing to changing yourself?

By shifting our thoughts, actions, words, perceptions, and choices, we transform our personal reality. These changes ripple outward, touching lives and contributing to a more conscious, harmonious, and healthy world.

Now, it's your turn. Enjoy the feeling of your mind strengthening and your heart opening as you do this practice.

Week Nine Practices

Between the stimulus and response there is a space. In that space is our power to choose our response. In our response lies our growth and our freedom.

VIKTOR E. FRANKL

1. Do the Check Your Heart, Change Your Thoughts Journaling Practice

Dedicate a separate notebook just for your CYH practice, or purchase *The Yogi's Way: Check Your Heart, Change Your Thoughts Awareness Journal* at TheYogisWay.com/thebook. You may also download and print a two-page PDF of this exercise from TheYogis Way.com/thebook. Whichever tool you choose, engage in the CYH journaling practice three times a week (every other day) for the next four weeks, the duration of this program.

If you are using your own blank notebook, set it up as follows. When filling it out, remember to look back to the previous forty-eight hours.

DATE: _____

1. **Ahimsa:** Nonviolence. Gentle and meaningful thoughts, words, actions.

    +

    −

    Action:

2. **Satya:** Be truthful all day to yourself and others.

   +

   −

   Action:

3. **Asteya:** Refrain from stealing. Honor other people's property, time, talents, and resources.

   +

   −

   Action:

4. **Brahmacharya:** Nourish relationships. See the light in all beings. Honor commitments. Engage in responsible sexual behavior.

   +

   −

   Action:

5. **Aparigraha:** Nongrasping. Let go of what you don't need. Practice generosity.

   +

   −

   Action:

6. **Saucha:** Cleanliness. Keep the space in your home and heart simple and clean.

   +

   −

   Action:

7. **Santosha:** Contentment. Rejoice in other people's successes. Be happy and grateful for what you have.

   +

–

Action:

8. **Tapas:** Fiery determination to live your purpose.

   +

   –

   Action:

9. **Svadhyaya:** Self-reflection, self-study with the purpose to understand rather than judge.

   +

   –

   Action:

10. **Ishvara pranidhana:** Surrender and trust. Do you allow life to happen as it does, or do you resist what is?

    +

    –

    Action:

Vedic philosophy is timeless because it describes realities that don't change. One of these realities is the way the mind works. The mind can take us into ditches every day, turning us toward food, people, entertainment, or media that harm us, depleting our life force. Or the mind can uplift us and align us with our gifts and potential. What makes the difference? You. You have a choice. Will you let your mind rule you, or will you become the chariot driver, actively choosing your thoughts and shaping your life?

2. Switch Up Your Other Journaling Practices

This week, we will scale back the Klesha Trigger Log to every other day instead of every day; from here on you'll do it three times a week until the end of the course. My suggestion is to sit with your journal every evening. One evening do the KTL and CYH practices, which will take fifteen to twenty minutes total. The next evening, write freely in your journal for approximately fifteen minutes.

As you journal, refrain from thinking too much. Connect to your heart and let the pen flow. Don't worry if your writing is messy or in half sentences. Let yourself write about whatever is present for you in the moment. Build a connection with your heart and with the ability to express what is arising within. This will help you cultivate presence as well as a connection with your feelings, experiences, intuition, and inner knowing.

Week Nine Daily Practice Sequence

Don't forget to include your joy date among your practices this week!

1. In My Own Hands: fifteen seconds
2. Optimal Breath practice: three minutes at the beginning of the day
3. All-Day Yoga
4. Sun Salutations with chakra awareness and mantras: fifteen to twenty minutes
5. Witness Meditation: six minutes
6. Savasana: five minutes
7. Journaling: five to ten minutes (reflecting on your practices)
8. Klesha Trigger Log and Check Your Heart, Change Your Thoughts: fifteen to twenty minutes every other day
9. Free Journaling: fifteen minutes on alternate days

Total daily practice time: approximately fifty to sixty minutes

Week Nine Mitra Meeting

What has been your experience of the CYH practice? What are you learning? How does it feel to replace harmful thoughts with nourishing ones? Have you had any realizations this week? Do you have any questions to go over with your mitras? Teachings to debate and discuss?

All we experience is preceded by mind, led by mind, made by mind. Speak or act with a corrupt mind and suffering follows as the wagon wheel follows the hoof of the ox. All we experience is preceded by mind, led by mind, made by mind. Speak or act with a peaceful mind and happiness follows like a shadow that never leaves.

Dhammapada (1.1–2)

Key Terms from Week Nine

Yamas: Ethical principles.
   Ahimsa: Nonviolence.
   Satya: Truth.
   Asteya: Nonstealing.
   Brahmacharya: Moderation.
   Aparigraha: Nongrasping.

Niyamas: Personal observances.
   Saucha: Cleanliness.
   Santosha: Contentment.
   Tapas: Discipline.
   Svadhyaya: Self-study.
   Ishvara Pranidhana: Surrender.

SELF-HEALING

The Medical Side of Yoga

The body is your temple.

B. K. S. IYENGAR

Why do some of us experience more anxiety than others? Why do some of us struggle more with anger or attachment than others? On this path, we are asked to love ourselves through all our fluctuating emotions, thoughts, sensations, and experiences. Where does the ability to practice self-love come from? Loving ourselves arises from understanding ourselves, a powerful step toward healing.

The science of Ayurveda offers deep insight into our unique constitution, which encompasses the biological forces affecting our physical and mental makeup. As we get to know our constitution — which we will in this chapter — we begin to comprehend how mental and physical imbalances are generated in our system and how to rectify those imbalances. We learn to work with our constitution instead of against it.

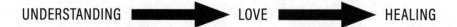

FIGURE 13: Understanding ourselves supports us in loving ourselves, which is a powerful step toward healing.

Yoga and Ayurveda were traditionally learned and practiced together, each complementing the other. Yoga is a spiritual science focused on self-realization, while Ayurveda is the science of self-healing. Together, they form a holistic approach where healing the mind and body serves as the foundation for spiritual growth — realizing who we truly are and living to our full potential.

In this chapter, I'll offer a brief overview of Ayurveda. Even a taste of these teachings can profoundly support your yoga journey.

The Sanskrit root *ayus* means "daily living." *Veda* is translated as "knowledge." *Ayurveda* means "the knowledge of daily living." Ayurveda is the art of living in harmony with the laws of nature. It is the knowledge of life beyond religion, dogma, and opinions. Yoga and Ayurveda come from the same source. They were both recorded in the Vedas approximately five thousand years ago. Ayurveda empowers individuals to discover how the forces of nature work within us. This deepens our knowledge of ourselves — our emotional tendencies and our triggers, as well as what foods, spices, climates, colors, aromas, and lifestyle choices throw us off-balance and which bring us back to center.

Though Ayurveda affects every aspect of our life, in this chapter, we will view it through three lenses. First, we will use it to gain insight into our mind's inclinations. Second, we will offer tips on improving our approach to diet and nutrition. (You will recall that nutrition is one of the pillars of the Yogi's Way.) And third, we will consider how understanding our nature can help us connect with and refine our svadharma. Each of these is a huge topic that merits a book in itself, but we will cover a few basics that you can begin to incorporate into your life this week.

The Prashna Upanishad describes a human being as a microcosm of the universe. Both are composed of prana — vital life force — that manifests in the form of earth, water, fire, air, and space. These five elements work in the environment and within our bodies and minds. The way these five elements are balanced within us differs from person to person and gives rise to our individual dosha, or constitution. For example, some of us have more fire in our system and are susceptible to sweating, fever, frustration, and anger. Some of us have more air in our constitution, which can manifest as dry skin, constipation, and anxiety. Those who have a dominance of the earth element within are more grounded than the rest of us. They are also susceptible to attachment and have a hard time letting things go that no longer serve them.

Learning about our constitution and those of the people close to us helps us understand and care for ourselves and others better. For example, when we are faced with people in whose constitution fire dominates, instead of judging them for their inclination toward anger, we remember that when this element is out of balance, anger is a natural tendency. Instead of spending time labeling the anger as something bad, we can assist them in bringing more water, earth, air, and space elements to their being — perhaps through a meal, a glass of water, a walk in nature on a cool day, or an encouragement to take a few cooling breaths before expressing their emotions to us or someone else.

Without this understanding of the elements within us, we may impulsively react and say something judgmental to someone experiencing an imbalance. When we know about the different constitutions and how they manifest in a person's behavior, we are aware of the underlying factors. This enables us to respond with empathy and compassion, offering solutions grounded in a deeper understanding.

Through an awareness of how we are susceptible to certain imbalances, we develop knowledge of small yet significant things we can shift in our daily life to regain and maintain balance. On this path, individuals are responsible for understanding how imbalances manifest from our daily living and for discovering — often through trial and error — how to regain and maintain equilibrium. *Balancing the five elements within is the basis of all Ayurvedic therapy.*

When I realized that my constitution is *vata*, which means I have a dominance of the air element within, it helped me be less judgmental toward myself when I struggle with anxiety. Those who have a dominance of the air element share this characteristic. The mind can get especially restless because earth is the element that we are most lacking. For us, grounding foods and yoga practices can be very effective when we are feeling unstable. In this manner, as we get to know our constitution, we can shift our lifestyle and yoga practices in subtle ways that make a difference.

Ayurveda consists of outer and inner therapies. Inner therapies include working with diet, herbs, breath, meditation, and Ayurvedic cleanses. Outer therapies include massage, exercise, and color, aroma, sound, and gem therapies.

The secret to radiant health, according to Ayurveda, is to recognize and accept our innate strengths and inclinations as well as our vulnerabilities and shortcomings. Our practice is to know ourselves and work *with* our nature, not against it. This is how we can love ourselves well. If we push ourselves in ways that are incompatible with our nature, we strain our body and mind.

Let's begin to understand ourselves better by discovering our constitution.

The Three Main Ayurvedic Constitutions

The precise way the five elements are balanced within each individual creates three main Ayurvedic *doshas*, or constitutions. These three doshas are called *vata*, *pitta*, and *kapha*.

Vata

For those with a vata-dominant constitution, air is the primary element, and ether is the secondary. *Va* is the Sanskrit root verb for "movement." *Vata* in Sanskrit literally means "wind." The vata constitution is known for having the qualities of wind and space, and the guiding principle is mobility — regulating activity in the body and mind.

Physical qualities: People who are vata dominant often have dry skin and hair, a thin build, a light and flexible body, and a dusky complexion. Vata individuals tend to be very short or very tall. They commonly experience digestive issues, such as constipation or abdominal gas. Emotional disturbances like stress or hostility can lead to nervous indigestion. Cold, windy, and dry conditions tend to unsettle them the most. Generally, vata individuals possess fragile health, despite their active nature. They thrive on movement and speed, yet they fatigue quickly and struggle with sustaining endurance.

Mental qualities: Individuals with a predominantly vata constitution possess agile and quick minds, characterized by frequent shifts in interests. They are often talkative, well-informed, and intellectual but can be absent-minded. While they may have a broad range of knowledge, they often lack expertise in a single subject. Vata types tend to be excitable, nervous, and restless, with minds that easily wander and wills that are often indecisive and unsteady. They embrace movement and change, showcasing remarkable adaptability and flexibility due to their sensitive and rapid-thinking minds. An excess of the air element, however, can lead to heightened anxiety, fearfulness, and insecurity.

Vata individuals excel as teachers and communicators, demonstrating proficiency in thinking and writing. Despite potential sensitivity to noise, many possess innate musical talents, reflecting their creative and artistic inclinations. While they can be sociable, the predominant air element may drive them toward solitude, as they have a heightened sensitivity to interpersonal interactions.

Sensory qualities: The senses of touch and hearing — which correspond to air and ether elements — are most significant for vata. Gold and greens are soothing colors for this constitution.

Balance for vata: Vata individuals benefit from eating warm, well-cooked, moist foods with sweet, sour, or salty tastes. They should avoid cold temperatures, minimize consumption of raw foods, refrain from eating too many beans, maintain a regular routine, and abide in a safe, warm, calm, quiet, and secure environment.

Imbalance for vata: Worry, fasting, lack of sleep, eating on the run, no routine, dry food, leftovers, no skin lubrication, cold weather, and repressing feelings foster imbalance in vata-dominant people.

Pitta

For those with a pitta constitution, fire is the primary element and water is secondary. *Pitta* comes from the Sanskrit word *tapa*, "to heat." It represents fire in the body and regulates body heat.

Physical qualities: Pitta individuals typically exhibit an average height and build. They have a robust appetite and thirst yet often maintain a stable weight. Their skin tends to be oily and vibrant, albeit prone to acne and rashes. Being fire types, they sweat easily and are inclined toward diarrhea because of their hot blood, making them susceptible to bruising and bleeding. Common health issues among pitta types include fevers, infections, and inflammations. They have a low tolerance for heat and bright light, preferring cool environments, water, and shade. Pitta individuals enjoy engaging in exercise and sports, showcasing moderate endurance. However, their competitive spirit often pushes them to the point of exhaustion.

Mental qualities: Pitta governs reason, intelligence, and discernment, enabling the mind to perceive and analyze. Individuals with a predominantly pitta constitution demonstrate exceptional concentration, organizational prowess, and firm principles. However, because of their sharp minds and fiery constitution, pitta imbalances may manifest as being opinionated, judgmental, or self-righteous, accompanied by irritability, frustration, anger, and a propensity for arguments. They may exhibit traits of aggressiveness and dominance.

Pitta types often excel in leadership roles, public speaking, scientific endeavors, legal professions, and politics, thriving on authority. Yet their determination may sometimes overshadow compassion, making it challenging for them to empathize with alternative perspectives. When properly directed, their resolute nature can lead to remarkable achievements.

Sensory qualities: Sight and taste, which correspond to fire and water, are most significant for pitta types. Blues and grays are soothing colors to pitta.

Balance for pitta: Keeping cool and avoiding excess heat, steam, and humidity are important for pitta individuals. They should stay away from excess oils, fried foods, caffeine, salt, alcohol, red meat, and overly hot spices. Fresh fruits and veggies, milk, cottage cheese, and whole grains should be emphasized in their diet. Pitta types do well when they get plenty of fresh air, trust their feelings, and express them in ways that support them and those around them.

Imbalance for pitta: Alcohol and spicy, sour, and salty foods create imbalance, as do tight clothes, hot climates, and repressing feelings.

Kapha

For people with a kapha constitution, the primary element is water and the secondary is earth. In Sanskrit, *ka* means "water," and *pha* means "flourish." Kapha governs form and substance and is responsible for weight, cohesion, and stability.

Physical qualities: Kapha individuals typically possess a large, robust frame and have thick, oily, and smooth skin, often accompanied by curly hair. They have hearty appetites and enjoy sound sleep, exhibiting a steady metabolism. Prone to accumulating mucus, they may suffer from conditions associated with excess weight or water retention, such as obesity, congestive disorders, edema, and benign tumors. While they prefer a sedentary lifestyle, they possess strong endurance and can accomplish significant tasks once motivated. Their strength lies in consistency and perseverance rather than speed or agility, though they may struggle with initiative and discipline.

Mental qualities: In the realm of the mind, kapha influences feelings, emotions, and the ability to retain form. Kapha individuals are characterized by mental tranquility and stability, often displaying emotional depth, romanticism, sentimentality, and a profound capacity for love, devotion, and loyalty. However, their emotional imbalances may manifest as possessiveness, greed, or depression. Although they may learn at a slower pace, kapha individuals retain information well. While not necessarily the most creative, they excel at materializing ideas into tangible form and establishing structures and institutions. Unlike vata types, they exhibit stamina and are adept at seeing tasks through to completion rather than initiating them. Kapha individuals tend to resist change but thrive in stable, accepting environments. They are known for their reliability and make excellent providers, as evidenced in their roles as dependable parents, partners, colleagues, and friends. Many kapha individuals also demonstrate culinary prowess, grounding their connection to the earth element and finding fulfillment in roles such as chefs, singers, healthcare providers, teachers, social workers, managers, or bankers.

Sensory qualities: Kapha relates to the senses of taste and smell, which correspond to water and earth. They like to eat sweets. Bitter and pungent tastes are balancing for them. Purple hues are soothing for kapha.

Balance for kapha: Kapha types do best when they get plenty of physical activity every day, minimize consumption of fat, and avoid iced food and drinks, sweets, and too much bread. They should eat foods that are warm, light, and dry, consuming enough complex carbs to sustain energy. Drinking plenty of fluids is important, as is emphasizing pungent, bitter, and astringent tastes, fresh veggies, herbs, and spices.

Imbalance for kapha: Long naps after meals create imbalance. So do consuming fatty foods and oils, overeating, denying the creative self, too much dependence on others, lack of exercise, and repressing feelings.

Which Is Your Constitution?

Complete the questionnaire below based on how you've felt for the most part over the course of your lifetime, not necessarily how you feel today. Select V (vata), P (pitta), or K (kapha) for each item.

1. **Physique**
   V Taller or shorter than average
   P Average in height, with a moderately developed physique
   K Broad, large, well-developed physique

2. **Weight**
   V Thin with prominent bones
   P Moderate weight
   K Heavy and tending toward overweight

3. **Hair**
   V Dry, curly, coarse, black, or dark brown
   P Red, light brown, blond, soft, fine, prone to premature graying or balding
   K Thick, oily, wavy, medium to dark brown

4. **Teeth**
    V   Crooked, large, protruding; receding gums
    P   Medium sized, yellowish; gums bleed easily
    K   Strong, straight, white

5. **Skin**
    V   Dry, rough, cool, brown, black
    P   Soft, oily, warm, red, yellowish
    K   Thick, oily, cool, pale, white

6. **Eyes**
    V   Small, dry, active
    P   Sharp, penetrating
    K   Big, with thick eyelashes

7. **Appetite**
    V   Variable, erratic — sometimes no appetite, sometimes very hungry
    P   Good, sharp, excessive; can digest large amounts of food
    K   Slow, steady; feels best with small quantities of food several times a day

8. **Elimination**
    V   Dry, hard; tendency toward constipation and gas
    P   Regular, soft; tendency toward diarrhea
    K   Large, heavy, oily

9. **Urine**
    V   Small amounts frequently
    P   Abundant, deep yellow, sometimes slight burning
    K   Moderate, concentrated

10. **Perspiration**
    V   Scanty, not much odor
    P   Profuse, strong odor
    K   Moderate

11. **Physical activity**
    V   Very active, fast; can tire or get distracted easily
    P   Moderate, efficient, perfectionistic; can get aggravated
    K   Lethargic, slow, deliberate, calm

12. **Mental activity**
    V   Restless, active, curious
    P   Aggressive, intelligent
    K   Calm, slow, receptive

13. **Learning style**
    V   Learns quickly, can forget easily
    P   Moderately quick
    K   Takes time but remembers well

14. **Emotional tendencies**
    V   Fearful, insecure, anxious
    P   Aggressive, irritable, jealous
    K   Attached, self-contented, greedy

15. **Immunity**
    V   Low; suffers minor illnesses often
    P   Moderate
    K   Rarely gets sick

16. **Disease patterns**
    V   Fatigue, nervous system issues, insomnia, dryness, arthritis

P   Fever, inflammation, infection, ulcers, skin conditions

K   Congestion, respiratory conditions, obesity

17. **Speech**

V   Talks a lot, shows enthusiasm

P   Argumentative, precise, convincing, direct

K   Slow, monotonous, low-pitched, rhythmic

18. **Social tendencies**

V   Insecure and nervous

P   Outgoing, assertive, accessible

K   More listening than speaking

19. **Concentration**

V   Easily distracted

P   Rarely distracted, intensely engaged

K   Moderate levels of concentration

20. **Truthfulness**

V   Will often harmlessly lie to avoid discomfort

P   Usually tells the truth

K   Never lies

21. **Willpower**

V   Weak; starts strong but often gives in

P   Moderate

K   Strong

22. **Mental tendencies**

V   Questions everything; creative

P   Discriminating, judging, suspicious

K   Logical, stable, reasonable

23. **Forgiveness**
   V   Forgives easily
   P   Takes a very long time to forgive
   K   Rarely upset, understanding

24. **Dreams**
   V   Flying, running, fearful
   P   Sharp, passionate, with imagery of sun, violence, colors
   K   Romantic, slow-moving; feature water

25. **Sleep**
   V   Scanty, interrupted
   P   Sound; requires less than other types
   K   Heavy, excessive

26. **Sex drive**
   V   Frequent desire, low stamina
   P   Moderate desire, passionate, dominating
   K   Cyclical, good stamina

27. **Work**
   V   Selfless; often volunteers
   P   Achievement oriented, especially with personal goals
   K   Procrastinates, takes time to complete projects

28. **Financial**
   V   Spends quickly and impulsively
   P   Spends moderately and methodically, enjoys luxuries
   K   Spends carefully, saves

Total: Vata _____ Pitta _____ Kapha _____

Most of us are a combination of two constitutions, or doshas. We have a dominant and a subdominant dosha: For example, you might be vata-pitta, pitta-vata, or kapha-pitta. If you feel a resonance with two doshas, that is normal. If your highest count and second highest count are not too far apart, then it is likely that you have a dominant and a subdominant dosha. If your highest count is higher by far than the other two, you likely have a dominant dosha.

It is always best to work with an Ayurvedic therapist or doctor to get a solid understanding of your constitution. For now, use your intuition along with the totals from the above questionnaire. What do you feel is your constitution? You will be surprised how often people are right about their constitution before they approach an Ayurvedic therapist or doctor for a full consultation.

The Three *Gunas*

Gunas is a Sanskrit word that means the energetic qualities or tendencies found in food, movement, meditation, and more. There are three main gunas:

- *Tamas:* Inertia
- *Rajas:* Activity
- *Sattva:* Harmony

All three gunas are present in every experience, yet they are constantly shifting, depending on how we respond to each situation. For example, if we can't peel ourselves away from our devices to go to the gym, tamas has taken the reins. If we overreact when a stranger gives us a seemingly unkind look, rajas becomes dominant. When we emerge from a beautiful hike in nature, we may experience the sattvic qualities of balance and joy.

The ways the gunas often manifest in each of the three constitutions is as follows.

Vata

- **Tamas:** Confusion, lack of direction, indecisiveness, sadness, grief
- **Rajas:** Hyperactivity, nervousness, fear, anxiety, ungroundedness
- **Sattva:** Clarity, creativity, lightness

Pitta

- **Tamas:** Anger, hatred, envy, jealousy
- **Rajas:** Aggressiveness, competitiveness, power, prestige
- **Sattva:** Knowledge, understanding, comprehension, recognition

Kapha

- **Tamas:** Deep confusion, depression, unconsciousness
- **Rajas:** Attachment, possessiveness, greed
- **Sattva:** Love, compassion, forgiveness

Understanding and working with the gunas can provide valuable insights into how we interact with the world and ourselves. By becoming aware of these energetic qualities and their influence on our thoughts, emotions, and behaviors, we can make more conscious choices to foster balance and well-being. For example, by recognizing when tamas, rajas, or sattva are dominant, we can adjust our activities, yoga practices, and diet to enhance overall harmony, which supports personal and spiritual development.

Ayurvedic Guidelines for Healthful Eating

Understanding your constitution — getting to know which foods, tastes, herbs, and spices work best for you — can help you cultivate inner equilibrium, leading to a healthy, vibrant life that also supports your journey toward spiritual growth and the realization of your purpose and potential. Before we go into some of those details, here is a list of basic Ayurvedic guidelines for healthful eating. You can bring these practices into your life this week.

- Eat in pleasant surroundings and in a relaxed state, avoiding rushing through your meal.
- Focus on the food while eating, minimizing heavy or complex conversations.
- Chew your food thoroughly to form a paste in the mouth, releasing digestive enzymes in the saliva to aid digestion.
- Practice moderation, consuming proper portions, and avoiding overeating.
- Eat on an empty stomach, waiting until the previous meal has been fully digested.
- Maintain regular mealtimes to promote healthy digestion.
- Incorporate variety in your diet to ensure a balanced nutritional intake.
- Enhance the flavor and digestibility of meals with Ayurvedic spices.
- Avoid processed, canned, frozen, and microwaved foods, as well as GMOs.
- Wash hands, face, mouth, and eyes after meals to support digestive health.
- Allow time for rest after lunch and consider a leisurely walk after dinner to aid digestion.
- Chew anise or fennel seeds after meals to aid digestion and freshen breath.

Rasas: The Six Tastes

Ayurveda recognizes six *rasas*, or tastes: sweet, sour, salty, pungent, bitter, and astringent. Each rasa is characterized by a specific set of dominant elements that create heat, coolness, dryness, or lightness.

Sweet

- **Elements:** Earth and water — cooling
- **Effect on doshas:** Decreases vata and pitta, increases kapha

Sour

- **Elements:** Earth and fire — warming
- **Effect on doshas:** Decreases vata, increases pitta and kapha

Salty

- **Elements:** Fire and water — warming
- **Effect on doshas:** Decreases vata, increases pitta and kapha

Pungent

- **Elements:** Air and fire — heating
- **Effect on doshas:** Decreases kapha, increases vata and pitta

Bitter

- **Elements:** Air and space — cooling
- **Effect on doshas:** Decreases pitta and kapha, increases vata

Astringent

- **Elements:** Air and earth — cooling, lightening, drying
- **Effect on doshas:** Decreases pitta and kapha, increases vata

Understanding your constitution enables you to discern which tastes are most beneficial for you. These are the rasas that promote balance for each dosha:

- **Vata:** Sweet, sour, salty
- **Pitta:** Sweet, bitter, astringent
- **Kapha:** Pungent, bitter, astringent

Food

Ayurveda views food as a means to balance the energy of prana in the body. The principles of Ayurvedic nutrition and cooking are vast and can be studied throughout one's lifetime. This week, let's delve into the fundamentals by exploring which foods and tastes to add or reduce in our diets. Now that you've been introduced to the beneficial tastes for your constitution, here are examples of foods that contain them and more details on the way each rasa's qualities affect each dosha.

Sweet

- **Foods:** Rice, milk, ghee, oil, bread, sugar, molasses, sweet fruits
- **Effect on doshas:** Balances vata and pitta but can increase kapha. It provides nourishment and grounding and soothes inflammation and dryness. Excess can lead to weight gain and congestion.

Sour

- **Foods:** Yogurt, cheese, vinegar, pickles, tomatoes, lemons, citrus fruits
- **Effect on doshas:** Balances vata but can increase pitta and kapha. It simulates digestion but can aggravate acidity and inflammation.

Salty

- **Foods:** Salt
- **Effect on doshas:** Balances vata but can increase pitta and kapha. Although it may initially stimulate kapha, its long-term effects can be counterproductive for this type, potentially leading to water retention and hypertension.

Pungent

- **Foods:** Chili peppers, ginger, black pepper, mustard, cloves, cinnamon, garlic, onions
- **Effect on doshas:** Balances kapha but can aggravate vata and pitta. For vata, small amounts can be OK if balanced with sweet, sour, or salty tastes.

Bitter

- **Foods:** Dark-green leafy veggies, Swedish bitters, broccoli, romaine, endive, celery, turmeric, citrus fruits
- **Effect on doshas:** Helps soothe and balance pitta; good for kapha as it reduces excess moisture and heaviness; can aggravate dryness and anxiety for vata.

Astringent

- **Foods:** Beans, lentils, tea, cabbage, cauliflower, greens, kiwifruit, apples, pomegranates, persimmons, cranberries
- **Effect on doshas:** Best for pitta and kapha as it helps control excess inflammation and moisture. Best avoided by vata as it can lead to dryness and constipation.

Week Ten Practices

1. Be the Medicine

Ultimately, on this path, your own awareness becomes your teacher and healer. What did you learn about the inclinations of your mind and body this week? Does this help you cultivate understanding and compassion for yourself? Write about this in your journal.

Food has a huge impact on our energy and is part of our daily lives. This is why nutrition is one of the pillars of the Yogi's Way. Try to bring the twelve Ayurvedic principles for eating (page 204) into your life this week as you shop for groceries and prepare food for yourself and your loved ones.

Now that you have an idea about your constitution, which of the six tastes can you incorporate more into your diet? Through which foods? If this is confusing, that's OK. It can take time to integrate all this information, and you may want to arrange a consultation with an Ayurvedic nutritionist to help you. In the meantime, trust your intuition to experiment with some changes in food choices and tastes while seeing how it feels to bring the basic principles of Ayurvedic eating into your life.

In Ayurvedic healing (as in all aspects of yoga), cultivating awareness is paramount. Imbalances are believed to stem from a lack of awareness, with physical ailments arising from external factors, such as diet and exposure to pathogens, while mental afflictions emerge from internal sources, like the accumulation of kleshas. To initiate your process of self-awareness regarding energy usage and toxin accumulation in your body, consider the following sets of questions.

Physical Toxins

- Do I consistently sleep well?
- Do I maintain a steady level of energy throughout the day?
- Are my digestion and elimination processes regular?
- Is my appetite consistently healthy?
- Is my skin in good condition?

Mental Toxins

- Am I able to relax both my mind and my body effectively?
- Do I engage in open communication with family, friends, and colleagues?

- When facing challenges or life disruptions, am I resilient in regaining balance?
- Are my relationships generally healthy and supportive?
- Do I prioritize self-care and allocate time for it?
- Do I frequently experience feelings of irritability or of calmness?

2. Ayurveda Awareness Journal

On any given day, toxins can build up through seemingly innocuous behaviors, like shallow breathing, reacting to a hurtful remark, or engaging in prolonged screen time. Maintaining a daily journal documenting activities, diet, and emotions can aid in fostering awareness, promoting self-healing, and facilitating self-realization. For the next three weeks, spend about three minutes each day tracking the following in your journal:

- Hours, time, and quality of sleep
- Digestive patterns
- Meal timings
- Diet changes
- Food sources and preparation methods
- Water intake
- Physical activity and meditation practices (duration and timing)
- Participation in other programs, therapies, or activities
- Energy fluctuations
- Overall emotional state

3. Understand. Love. Heal.

Reviewing the "Which Is Your Constitution?" questionnaire on page 197, try to determine the constitution of one or two people closest to you — perhaps a family member or a mitra. Applying what you learned in this chapter, what is something you discovered about them that causes you to feel more empathetic toward them? Can you think of ways to better care for them?

4. Explore Your Svadharma

When you bring forth what is within you, what you bring forth will save you. When you do not bring forth what is within you, what you do not bring forth will destroy you.

GOSPEL OF THOMAS (70)

When you bring forth what is within you, what you bring forth will save the world.

BHAGAVAD GITA

In Week Five, we released the labels and stories that limit us and began to connect with the spacious dimension that exists at the center of our being — a reflection of our limitless potential. Then, in Week Six, we planted seeds in that space of confidence and worth. Let's take this further. From the spacious, nonjudgmental seat of consciousness, we'll explore our svadharma, either discovering it for the first time or refining or updating it. Remember, it's OK to play with our personality, to experiment with different inclinations. We are not fixed beings. Things change, and we can let them.

First, send yourself this wish: *May I be genuinely happy.* Remember, wanting happiness is not selfish. Review your motivation from Week One. We are not trying to acquire something from the world. Instead, we are exploring the possibility of experiencing genuine happiness by giving our svadharma *to* the world.

Think of someone you love dearly. Close your eyes. From your heart, send this person the wish *May you be truly happy.* Naturally, you send the wish with great affection, because you love this person.

Now, with this same affection, send that wish to yourself again: *May I be genuinely happy.**

The Brihadaranyaka Upanishad advises us to get in touch with our deepest desires. We are encouraged to allow one or two of our strongest desires to shape our life. If we have many goals and dreams, our energy gets scattered, and we may run ourselves thin. Consider the power of one large river moving in a certain direction as opposed to the energy of many small rivers. If you have one or two major goals, decision-making becomes easier: Would this choice move me closer to my goal or not?

> *You are what your deep, driving desire is.*
> *As your desire is, so is your will.*
> *As your will is, so is your deed.*
> *As your deed is, so is your destiny.*

BRIHADARANYAKA UPANISHAD (4.4.5)

Remember, Ayurveda teaches us to understand our nature and honor it by living according to it. To explore your svadharma, complete the following sentences in your journal. Dig deep. There are no restrictions. Have fun with the exercise below.†

First, reflect on the past:

- The most joyful moment I experienced in the past week was...
- The most joyful moment I experienced in the past month was...
- The most joyful moment I experienced in the past year was...

---

*   I learned this practice in a live teaching with meditation teacher Douglas
       Veenhof in 2015. See DouglasVeenhof.com.
†   I learned the first three items in this exercise from Douglas Veenhof.

- The things I've accomplished in my life that are most meaningful to me are…

Next, consider where your desires are pulling you. What are your passions, the things that light a fire within you and that you'd love to explore in your life? For example, perhaps you are drawn to design, music, theater, medicine, science, community building, architecture, art, healing, exercise, animals, and/or travel. Now, complete these prompts:

- I am naturally drawn to…
- I would love to learn more about…
- I would love to acquire skills in…
- I would love to take a course in…
- I would love to apprentice with…

Next, read the statements you wrote out loud. How does it feel in your body to acknowledge and hear yourself say them?

Wherever you are right now is where you're meant to be. Rejoice in the fact that you are making space to connect with your innate capacity, interests, and gifts — your svadharma. Refrain from letting the mind go to feelings of guilt or shame if you feel off track with your svadharma. Practice intelligent regret as opposed to dysfunctional guilt.

The Japanese have a concept called *ikigai*: that which gives your life meaning. Ikigai is found at the intersection of four rules:

1. Do what you love.
2. Do what you're good at.
3. Do what the world needs.
4. Do what you can be paid for.

In considering the four rules, notice where there is overlap for you (see figure 14). Make a note of any insights in your journal.

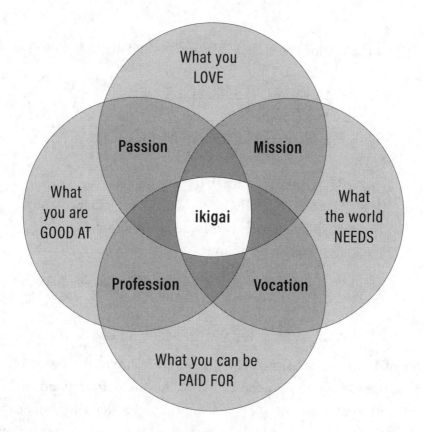

FIGURE 14: Ikigai.

In your journal, also reflect on your svadharma. Is this a time in your life to discover, update, or refine it? How do you feel about it? What are your deepest desires? Do you need more time in the not knowing? This is OK too. Write freely about this for ten minutes or more.

Week Ten Daily Practice Sequence

Remember to include your joy date in this week's practices.

1. In My Own Hands: fifteen seconds
2. Optimal Breath practice: three minutes at the beginning of the day

3. All-Day Yoga

4. Sun Salutations with chakra awareness and mantras: fifteen to twenty minutes

5. Witness Meditation: six minutes

6. Savasana: five minutes

7. Journaling: five to ten minutes (reflecting on the practices above)

8. Ayurveda Awareness Journal: three minutes

9. Klesha Trigger Log and Check Your Heart, Change Your Thoughts: fifteen to twenty minutes every other day

10. Free Journaling: fifteen minutes on alternate days

Total daily practice time: approximately fifty to sixty minutes

Week Ten Mitra Meeting

Share what you've learned about your constitution with your mitras. Does knowing your constitution help you to understand yourself better? In what ways? Does this help you foster self-love? Any shifts to your diet? How did this week's teachings affect your grocery shopping, food preparation, and eating experiences? How are you feeling about your svadharma? What did you do for your joy date this week? Maybe it was something food related, like treating yourself to a delicious and healthy meal or going to a library, browsing the Ayurvedic cookbooks, and choosing one that inspired you.

Key Terms from Week Ten

Ayurveda: The knowledge of balanced daily living, which leads to self-healing.

Dosha: The body's constitution. There are three main types: vata, the dosha of wind; pitta, the dosha of heat; and kapha, the dosha of wetness.

Gunas: The three energetic qualities found in nature, including in food: tamas, the guna of inertia; rajas, the guna of activity; and sattva, the guna of harmony.

Rasas: The six tastes that can create balance or imbalance within the body: sweet, sour, salty, pungent, bitter, and astringent.

MEDITATION

Develop Concentration, Stability, and Clarity

*All of humanity's problems stem from man's inability
to sit quietly in a room alone.*

BLAISE PASCAL

Our journey with meditation began in Week Two when we became present with the quality of our breath. As we developed the skill of breath awareness, we expanded this ability to become aware of emotions. We identified our major kleshas and began to familiarize ourselves with what triggers them. Since Week Four, we have practiced observing ourselves from the quiet, spacious, non-judgmental seat of the witness.

This week, we will delve deeper into the art of meditation. Today, the term *meditation* is used in many different ways. In the Vedic tradition, meditation means something very specific: one-pointed concentration. A study from Harvard happiness experts found a direct correlation between happiness and a focused mind. According to the study, participants spent nearly 47 percent of their waking hours with their minds wandering. When people were thinking about something other than what they were doing, they felt less happy. Even when distracted by pleasurable thoughts, participants were less happy than those who were fully present with their current activities. The study's author, Matthew Killingsworth, concluded that this research supports a key principle found in many spiritual traditions: Being present is essential for happiness.

After reviewing ten years of research, the American Medical Association concluded that meditation is as effective as medication in treating depression, anxiety, and visceral pain. Meditation has a profound impact at the molecular level on the endocrine system and even on our genetics.

Meditation orchestrates the simultaneous release of the neurotransmitters dopamine, serotonin, oxytocin, and endorphins. Dopamine enhances pleasure, reward, and focus. Serotonin reduces tension and stress, promoting a calm and relaxed mind. Oxytocin fosters feelings of pleasure, security, and contentment while reducing fear and anxiety. Endorphins, known for producing the "runner's high," create exhilaration and decrease pain and stress. This synchronized release of neurotransmitters is something that no single drug can do. Meditation does it without dangerous side effects.

In contemporary times, meditation can be difficult for us all. Our minds are often racing and hyperactive, in part because of our incessant exposure to media and the digital realm. We have come to crave stimuli, which impedes our ability to sustain focus on a chosen object. As highlighted in the previously cited Harvard study, nearly half the population experiences a wandering mind at any given moment. Consequently, our productivity suffers across various domains, be they educational settings, workplaces, or the home environment. What can we do to turn this around?

When the impulse arises to reach for a distraction — whether that be your phone or an unhealthy snack — take a moment to pause, breathe deeply, and refocus on the task at hand. Each time you resist the allure of these distractions, you strengthen your willpower and enhance your ability to meditate.

In this chapter, we will set the stage for deeper meditation experiences. Then, we will add a six-minute Consciousness Meditation practice to our daily six-minute Witness Meditation practice.

Delving into the Three Gunas

Last week, you were introduced to the three gunas, the energetic qualities or tendencies found in food as well as in our mind and body. To review, the three main gunas are:

- **Tamas:** Nature's destructive energy: inertia, heaviness, lethargy
- **Rajas:** Nature's creative energy: activity, movement, change
- **Sattva:** Nature's preserving energy: harmony, balance, wholesomeness

Chapter 14 of the Bhagavad Gita urges us to understand that everything in nature, including our own mind, is in constant flux among these three states. Every day, we experience these three states. No matter which one dominates in the moment, the Gita implores us not to long for something different. As a witness, we stand aside and watch the three states arise, abide, and dissolve while being accepting and judgment-free. Just like nature itself, it is the nature of our mind to move among these three states. Understanding this helps us stay rooted in the witness consciousness, which is free of the need to analyze, grasp, or resist. As the witness, we can truly let the river of emotions, thoughts, and experiences flow without becoming overwhelmed.

Remember, as the witness, we don't label any of these three states as good, bad, better, or worse. They are simply a part of the human experience. Someone in a sattvic state, for example, is calm, joyful, balanced, and content, but becoming attached to this state or yearning for it when it is absent can be stressful and restrictive. We may become avoidant of anger or attachment when it is present and deprive ourselves of the opportunity to heal and be whole. In a rajasic state, to take another example, we act. This can be a great thing. However, if we become attached to moving all the time or to clinging to the results of our actions, it can also be a source of bondage. And the third guna, tamas, may sound like a negative state, but allowing ourselves to rest is compulsory for a healthy and creative lifestyle.

The key to abiding in witness consciousness is understanding that it is natural to experience these three states even within the span of one meditation. When you begin to meditate, you might start in a rajasic state, feeling restless. As you take deep breaths and allow your body and mind to rest, you may move to a tamasic state of relaxation. By the end of the session, you might find yourself in a sattvic state of balance and clarity. The trick is not to identify ourselves with our present-moment thoughts, emotions, and actions. Who we truly are is something much more profound: the infinite field of possibility that the witness reflects.

In neuroscience and physiology, parallels can be drawn between the three gunas and polyvagal theory, which was introduced by the psychologist and neuroscientist Dr. Stephen Porges in 1994. This theory is based on the autonomic nervous system, which comprises the sympathetic and parasympathetic branches. These branches orchestrate our physiological responses — similar to the dynamics of rajas, tamas, and sattva in Ayurvedic and yogic philosophy (see figure 15).

Primarily situated in the spinal cord, the sympathetic branch mirrors rajas, mobilizing us for action by releasing adrenaline and other neurotransmitters that instigate the body's fight-or-flight response. The parasympathetic branch includes the vagus nerve, which has two distinctive pathways: the ventral and the dorsal pathways. The ventral vagal pathway, similar to sattva, creates a sense of harmony by sending our system cues of safety, nourishment, and joy, fostering relaxation and healthy social connections. Likewise, healthy, attuned interpersonal relationships enhance vagal tone, as do mindful movement, breathing, and meditation practices. This all helps us move through the world with more calm, ease, self-regulation, and resilience. In contrast, the dorsal vagal pathway, similar to tamas, responds to fatigue or danger by ushering us into a protective, immobilized state, rendering movement sluggish or the body inert. In the case of a threat to life, the dorsal pathway can shut down awareness through dissociation or fainting. How quickly we move into dorsal activation is contingent on our past experiences.

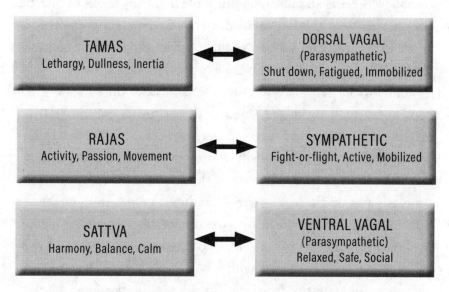

FIGURE 15: Polyvagal and Ayurvedic theories.

Over the years, while raising my daughter, there have been many times when I've been cherishing a rare moment of solitude, only to feel a deep urge to lie down and rest. I could succumb to self-judgment and tell myself I "should" get up and go for a run, practice asana, or go meet with friends whom I haven't seen for months. Yet I've come to realize that my body enters a natural tamasic or dorsal state because it needs to. Rather than interpreting this as laziness, I recognize it as an essential time for rejuvenation and the gathering of strength.

Listening to our body's call for rest is a vital step toward self-care and replenishment, aligning us with what's truly needed in the moment. When we honor this period of rest, we eventually transition from a tamasic or dorsal state into a sattvic or harmonious vagal state, feeling refreshed and balanced. When the time is right, we naturally progress into a rajasic or sympathetic state, ready to engage in activity once more. Understanding this natural process is essential for our overall well-being and for designing a life that truly meets our needs. In my experience, this has entailed stretching out of my comfort zone and learning to ask for support so that I can indeed take care of myself while navigating the responsibilities of parenthood.

Individuals may also shift into the tamasic or dorsal state when confronted with perceived threats. These threats can range from life-threatening experiences, such as a severe car accident that causes one to black out, to emotionally distressing events, like an adult relationship that triggers someone's childhood trauma. After some time, the person in the car wreck gradually comes to their senses, transitioning into the rajasic or sympathetic state, where they gather the energy to address the aftermath of the incident. Later that evening, after relaxing at home with a book, this person may begin to enter into the sattvic or vagal state, feeling safe and calm.

Similarly, the person who's been emotionally triggered may initially enter the panic-driven fight-or-flight or sympathetic state, characterized by symptoms like a racing heart, shortness of breath, and trembling hands. Overwhelmed by the intensity, they may then shift into the tamasic or dorsal state, withdrawing into a corner, disconnected from their surroundings. With time, they may seek support from friends, employ relaxation techniques, or find solace in nature, all of which help regulate the nervous system and facilitate a transition toward the ventral vagal state of sattvic peace and well-being.

Similar to the teachings of yoga and Ayurveda, in polyvagal theory, the three states — ventral vagal, sympathetic, and dorsal vagal — are not inherently good or bad. Instead, they represent adaptive strategies that our nervous system naturally employs in response to various environmental cues and internal states. Each state serves a specific function and can shift in response to changing circumstances. It's essential to recognize that experiencing each state is a normal part of being human.

I offer this basic overview of polyvagal theory to emphasize the importance of accepting our present-moment experiences wholeheartedly. Acceptance is the key to meditation. This entails accepting a moment as it is without wishing it to be different. Resistance to the present moment is futile because the moment is already happening. We can't change it. Our power lies in changing how we respond to the moment. When the moment is painful, rather than closing the heart to what is present, we strive to keep our heart open. As we've experienced in previous chapters, complete acceptance of our circumstances catalyzes transformation, while resistance only perpetuates the circumstance. By letting go of resistance and accepting what is, we naturally liberate adaptive energies and creativity.

A Deeper Dive into Meditation

In Week Four, we explored the analogy of the mind as a sea: The surface is often tumultuous and constantly shifting, while the depths are calm, still, and expansive. This week we will observe both the surface movements of the mind (in our review of the six-minute Witness Meditation from Week Four) and the deeper, unchanging dimension of consciousness (in the new, six-minute Consciousness Meditation).

In the Witness Meditation, we close our eyes and focus on the space behind our forehead, which mirrors the vastness of consciousness. This space is beginningless, endless, and boundless. We become a witness to any thought, emotion, sensation, or experience that arises in this space. Remember, the witness is neutral, remaining nonjudgmental and free from labeling emotions, thoughts, or experiences as good, bad, right, or wrong. As the watcher, we allow all experiences to unfold — pain, joy, confusion, clarity — without the mind's usual tendency to grasp, resist, compare, or judge.

Everything that arises in the space of consciousness is transient. Every thought, emotion, sensation, and experience appears, remains for a while, and then dissolves. Many of these thoughts and emotions are repetitive and deplete our energy. We have a choice: We can pay attention to them or not.

In this week's Consciousness Meditation, we shift our attention from the stream of thoughts, emotions, sensations, and experiences to consciousness itself. For six minutes each day, we will let the mind rest on this expansive presence, unchanging amid the ebb and flow of our energy and encounters.

Remember, consciousness is a field of pure potentiality. This infinite field of possibility is what yogis refer to as "the true Self" and the underlying reality of the world. It is a source of energy, love, and healing. Rather than getting caught up in all that changes, we learn to anchor ourselves in this unchanging dimension, preparing to navigate life's ups and downs with a steady and expansive awareness. Instead of getting overwhelmed by the clouds that pass by, we maintain a connection with the sky.

I live in the unchanging. I live in the sky, not the clouds.

SRI NISARGADATTA MAHARAJ

We spend our whole lives on the fleeting story — this body,
this mind — and no time on the source.

SRI RAMANA MAHARSHI

Spiritual guides across the globe inhabit dual realms simultaneously: the changing and the eternal. Anchored in the timeless, they dwell in eternal presence, accessing profound love and wisdom. They bring this into the changing dimension and become agents of healing and insight. Developing such a skill requires patience and a motivation to give, love, and serve. Every being has the capacity to dwell in both realms. This week's Consciousness Meditation prepares you to embrace the world with fervor and love fiercely while remaining rooted in the infinite. Being connected to this underlying field of possibility will help you cultivate a calm, spacious, and resilient mind as you navigate life's inevitable vicissitudes.

Week Eleven Practices

1. Meditation Prep

The following nine steps are practices that ready the mind for meditation, based on topics covered in this book. This Meditation Prep is meant to feel natural and supportive, not burdensome. As you become familiar with it, you will be able to go through these nine steps seamlessly in about three minutes. After that comes the Witness Meditation from Week Four (page 85), which leads into this week's Consciousness Meditation.

1. **Physical space.** Make sure your space is clean and free of clutter. Let this sacred area be device-free. If possible, choose a space where there is minimal outdoor noise. As much as you can, keep the environment comfortable — not

too hot or cold, with fresh air and natural light. Wear pleasant clothes that are light and loose. Be comfortable in your body — not starving and not too full. Feel free to create your own rituals, such as taking a shower, wearing a special clean outfit, and/or lighting a candle before you begin.

2. **Posture.** Sit on a chair or on the ground. If you are sitting on the floor, have a cushion or pillow to sit on. Elevating the hips a bit higher than the knees encourages length in the spine. Relax the hips toward the earth and lift the heart up to the sky. Relax your shoulder blades downward and breathe into the length of your spine. A well-aligned spine helps blocked energy at the base of the spine rise to our awareness.

3. **Breath.** Establish a slow, steady diaphragmatic breath, as you do in the Optimal Breath practice. Unless your nose is congested because of a cold or allergies, breathe through the nostrils. Use the next few breaths to relax your body. Draw the breath to any area that feels tense while maintaining length in the spine. If this is painful for any reason, rest your back against a wall.

4. **Turning inward.** Acknowledge that we have a human tendency to rely on things outside of ourselves for happiness: *Only when I get that job, relationship, house, et cetera, will I be happy.* In your mind, loosen the grip on something that you depend on outside of yourself for your happiness. As the grasp loosens, energy is freed. Direct that energy inward to rouse insight and creative energies that are ready to surface.

5. **Motivation.** Remind yourself that you are here to awaken

dormant energy so you have more love and wisdom to share in your unique ways. Bring in your personalized motivation from Week One here. Feel free to mentally refine or rewrite it.

6. **Blessings.** Depending on your faith and what resonates with you, ask for blessings from your guides, a higher power, or your higher Self. Visualize yourself receiving these blessings and feel yourself and your practice being blessed. Express gratitude for these blessings.

7. **I AM.** Remember that you are pure potential. On a subatomic level, your body is 99.9 percent empty space. Because you are empty of any fixed quality, you can become anything to fulfill your highest potential.

8. **Visualization.** Visualize the highest version of yourself. How does this self think, talk, act, move through the world? Picture yourself in detail. Let yourself dream. Remember, neuroplasticity gives the brain a remarkable capacity for forging new connections and pathways. Through visualization, we can actively reshape the brain's connectivity and enhance its performance. When you envision your best self, the mind is primed to take steps to make that vision a reality by leveraging the brain's adaptive capabilities.

9. **Gratitude.** Give thanks for your life and for all that you have.

2. Twelve-Minute Meditation Practice

Witness Meditation: Noticing What Changes

Set your timer for six minutes. As you breathe smoothly and deeply, close your eyes, connect with your third eye, and see the vast space behind your forehead. Become a witness to any thoughts, emotions, sensations, and experiences that arise in this space. Watch them come and go, flowing like a river. Let the mind express itself freely. Be lucidly awake to every thought, emotion, sensation, or experience that emerges. Watch each one arise, abide, and dissolve. Notice how each thought, emotion, and sensation is temporary.

When we are present with ourselves at this level, we become aware of what thoughts and emotions are alive for us in the moment. This helps us understand what is important to us. It also reveals repetitive patterns that may be harmful, making it clear which kleshas are affecting us so that we can address them in future practices.

The witness is a bridge to consciousness, as both remain undisturbed by passing thoughts, emotions, and experiences — like sunlight, which remains unchanged whether it falls on mud or clear water.

Consciousness Meditation: Noticing the Unchanging

Again, set your timer for six minutes. Close your eyes. Instead of paying attention to your present-moment thoughts, emotions, sensations, and experiences, focus on the space behind your forehead where all these phenomena arise, abide, and dissolve. Get to know this space. Notice that it is beginningless and endless. Whatever comes and goes here, the space itself is unaffected, undisturbed, undefended, and unchanging. Rest your mind on the infinite, eternal, unchanging presence of consciousness. Connect with this deepest, most boundless and liberated part of yourself. Every day become more familiar with consciousness, a primal source of energy, healing, love, and insight.

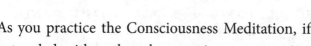

As you practice the Consciousness Meditation, if your mind gets entangled with a thought, emotion, or experience and you lose touch with the background of consciousness, try these tips:

- Take a deep breath. Refrain from judging yourself; instead, be glad you noticed. This is a win. Let the thought go and return to the vast field of consciousness. Each time you feel gripped by a thought, emotion, or experience, breathe deeply and use this mantra: *Release, return, rest.* Every day, you will be able to return and rest your attention for longer periods on the underlying, unchanging dimension of consciousness. Gradually, you will become more familiar with this changeless reality. This spacious realm is the quantum field of pure potentiality. To be aware of and yoked to this dimension *is* yoga.
- Another option if you find yourself caught up in an emotion or thought is to remember your essence: *I am light* or *I am divine.* These affirmations can serve as mantras to help you release, return, and rest your mind on the expansive field of consciousness. Remember, you are not your transient thoughts and emotions. You are something much more profound — the infinite, radiant soul who can direct your awareness with compassion and wisdom.
- It is possible — especially when an individual has gone through severe and unresolved trauma — that closing one's eyes to meditate can induce feelings of anxiety, fear, and the reexperience of past traumas. If this is the case for you or any of your mitras, it is best to meditate in a group where a safe space has been established and there is a qualified teacher

facilitating the experience. You can also try to meditate with your eyes open. Find a soft downward gaze by choosing a place on the ground to rest your eyes and see if your experience is more comfortable.

If you choose to continue with this meditation after completing the book, you may find that the Consciousness Meditation becomes particularly interesting. When we open ourselves to the eternal and infinite, remarkable things begin to unfold. You may connect with a loved one who has passed, a part of yourself deeply tucked away, or a nugget of insight that changes the trajectory of your life. Over time, you may want to extend your sessions, sitting in Consciousness Meditation for longer periods.

3. Self-Reflection

Since Week Two, you have been keeping a log of what triggers your kleshas. As we've explored in this chapter, emotional triggers often precipitate a shift into a sympathetic or rajasic state, experienced as increased heart rate, rapid breathing, heightened alertness, sweating, muscle tension, emotional intensity, and dilated pupils. Look over your Klesha Trigger Log and reflect on your experiences during such moments. In your journal, answer the following questions:

- What do you tend to experience in your body, mind, and heart when you are triggered?
- What patterns do you notice from the log that you've been keeping?

Moreover, consider and write down what strategies and practices help you return to a state of calmness and safety, characterized by vagal or sattvic qualities. You might find that returning to All-Day Yoga helps when you're feeling overstimulated. Whether

it's indulging in a warm bath, talking with a friend, walking in nature, chanting mantra, moving your body, or immersing yourself
in certain meditative yogic practices, document the techniques that
resonate most deeply with you.

Additionally, journal about your encounters with the dorsal or
tamasic states — the moments when you feel withdrawn, fatigued,
or disconnected from your surroundings. When you are in this
state, what practices or strategies help you the most? For instance,
sitting under the sun or listening to mantra may help when you feel
depleted or disconnected. By acknowledging and examining these
experiences, we continue to empower ourselves to navigate our
inner landscape with insight and resilience.

Finally, in your journaling, reflect on the process of shifting the
five samskaras you identified in the Guard Your Gates practice in
Week Seven (page 147).

Week Eleven Daily Practice Sequence

Don't forget to include your weekly joy date as part of your Week
Eleven practices.

You can integrate the Meditation Prep into the Optimal Breath
practice at the start of your day. This will set a meditative and spiritual tone to your entire day and all the practices that follow. Ideally,
follow the Meditation Prep with Sun Salutations, the twelve-minute
meditation, and Savasana for a forty-minute practice. If you need to
do the twelve-minute meditation practice at a separate time, start the
Meditation Prep before beginning your twelve-minute meditation.

Morning Practice (forty to forty-five minutes)

1. In My Own Hands: fifteen seconds
2. Meditation Prep (page 225), including Optimal Breath
   practice: six minutes

3. Sun Salutations with chakra awareness and mantras: fifteen to twenty minutes
4. Witness Meditation followed by Consciousness Meditation: six minutes each
5. Savasana: five minutes
6. Journaling: five minutes (reflecting on above practices)
7. All-Day Yoga

Evening Practice (twenty to twenty-five minutes):

1. Ayurveda Awareness Journal: three minutes
2. Klesha Trigger Log and Check Your Heart, Change Your Thoughts: fifteen to twenty minutes every other day
3. Free Journaling: fifteen minutes on alternate days

Total daily practice time: approximately sixty to seventy minutes

Week Eleven Mitra Meeting

Share with your mitras about the expansion of your meditation practice. How did the Meditation Prep impact your practice? Did it add a deeper dimension? How was your twelve-minute meditation practice this week? What is it like to be fully present and open to all that arises in the field of consciousness (Witness Meditation)? What is it like to give your full attention to consciousness itself (Consciousness Meditation)? Finally, take a moment to reflect on how you are feeling about your practices and life overall right now.

> *Wisdom says I am nothing.*
> *Love says I am everything.*
> *Between the two, my life flows.*
>
> SRI NISARGADATTA MAHARAJ

Key Terms from Week Eleven

Meditation: One-pointed concentration.

Autonomic nervous system: The part of your nervous system that controls unconscious functions, like your heartbeat and blood pressure.

Polyvagal theory: The theory that the autonomic nervous system's sympathetic and parasympathetic branches (particularly the vagus nerve in the latter) orchestrate our physiological responses.

Dorsal vagus: The pathway of the vagus nerve that resembles tamas; immobilizing.

Sympathetic: The branch of the autonomic nervous system that mirrors rajas; mobilizing.

Ventral vagus: The pathway of the vagus nerve that is similar to sattva; promotes harmony, safety, joy.

WEEK TWELVE

SERVICE AND CELEBRATION

Generate Daily Doses of Joy

*Peace is not something you wish for; it's something you make,
something you do, something you are, and something you give away.*

JOHN LENNON

It's not what we do that is most important. It's how we do the things we do. One of the most potent teachings of the Bhagavad Gita is to give 100 percent of our energy and attention to our present-moment actions without being concerned about the outcome. Chapter 2 of the Gita states: "Detached from results, put yourself wholeheartedly in the action. Be indifferent and unattached to the outcome" (2.47–48).

Thinking about outcome distracts us from the action itself. Not only does the quality of the act suffer, a mind that is preoccupied with results will always be anxious and stressed. This timeless wisdom text challenges us: Can we give ourselves fully to the present moment without worrying about the results of our actions? For example, can we enjoy the journey of working through harmful thoughts and emotions without being attached to an outcome, such as everlasting peace? There is a profound satisfaction we can experience by giving ourselves fully to each moment. It's so enriching to be completely present that the outcome ceases to matter as much. Ironically, when our mind and energy are fully immersed in the present moment, we experience the best results. This is why the saying goes, "Enjoy the journey. Don't worry about the destination." Peace is only available in the now. We can embody it now, in our willingness to give ourselves wholeheartedly to this moment.

Underlying our actions there exists the unchanging dimension of consciousness. Remember, the purpose of yoga is to be united with this eternal and infinite space. Since Week Four, we have been getting familiar with the seat of consciousness, rooting ourselves in the changeless dimension that underlies the world of change. What is your experience of this dimension? Do you experience it like the quantum physicists do, as a field of pure potentiality? Or, like Jesus, as a peace that passeth all understanding? Or, like the Buddhists, as emptiness or openness? Or, like the mystics, as love? Continue your explorations of what the Chandogya Upanishad calls "the Land of No Change." When we become familiar with this dimension, we can understand what is likely the Gita's most celebrated teaching: "Having made yourself alike in pain and pleasure, profit and loss, victory and defeat, engage in your great work" (2.38).

As I refine my svadharma, meditating on consciousness makes me more daring. I'm willing to try new things and tread unfamiliar territory because I'm in touch with the part of myself that is unaffected, undisturbed, and undamageable, whatever the outcome of my actions may be. This has helped me to see my life as an experiment.

For example, my daughter is in elementary school, and a couple of years ago, I developed a strong interest in bringing yoga and Ayurveda to children. Even though I had spent my career teaching adults, I made a switch. I studied the art of teaching yoga to kids and then began teaching at her school once a week. It was hard. Working with children required learning an entirely new set of skills. I didn't know if I would fail or succeed, if I'd be met with criticism or praise, if the classes would be horrible or wonderful. But I went for it. I knew that whatever the outcome, my essential nature of infinite space, possibility, and love would remain untouched. Perhaps I would love teaching children. Perhaps I would realize it was not something I wanted to pursue. Either way, there is freedom from being anxious about the results.

After a few weeks of teaching at the school for free, the administration helped me secure a grant to teach grades K–6 once a week for six months. My prayers were answered. I was grateful for this chance. Some classes were extremely difficult. A few of the kids wouldn't stop talking. I felt I had to speak over them, as there was a consistent background chatter going on among certain children in the classroom. I tried many tactics to get the class to quiet down so I could present a teaching. I would come home exhausted and bewildered. I had no idea how difficult it could be to get a group of kids to listen. I worried that the school's teachers and administrators, who sometimes peeked into my classes, would see me as a failure.

One day, when I was feeling defeated, I remembered that teaching from the Gita: to give 100 percent while letting go of the results of our actions.

That night, I told myself that I would give myself wholeheartedly to the children and not worry about the results. I decided to let go of any lessons I had planned for them and to teach from a place of pure presence and receptivity to whatever practice would best serve the children in each moment. Shortly thereafter I also reached out to seasoned teachers and learned some new and fun methods to get the children's attention and to calm down a rowdy classroom. I tried again and again. Some classes were still difficult. Other classes felt like a miracle. The children quieted, listened, and happily engaged in the movement, breathing, and mindfulness practices. I would step out of the room feeling amazed at how well things were going.

The weeks went on like this. I realized that when a class went well, I couldn't get attached to that outcome, because the next week

238 THE YOGI'S WAY

that same class could be my greatest challenge. When a class was difficult, I wouldn't let myself get attached to that either and allow my mind to become upset or frustrated, because I knew that this, too, would pass. The next week, the most difficult class from the previous week would go beautifully.

Isn't this a microcosm of life? Some days feel hard, like we are walking through mud, and everything that could go wrong does. Other days feel easeful, with pure joy and sweetness all around. The Gita is teaching us that the ups and downs of life won't stop. There is so much out there that we don't have control over. But *we* can change. *We* can be OK whether we sail smoothly through a challenge or fall flat on our face. *We* can be OK even if we have to pick ourselves up again and again. We can be in touch with that boundless, eternal part of ourselves that is a constant source of energy and love. Whatever happens in life, whatever we are given, and whatever is taken away from us, the underlying reality is a field of possibility and love. If we can stay anchored here, we can get through praise, criticism, profit, loss, joy, pain, success, and failure. In fact, these words cease to hold importance, because if we are rooted in consciousness, nothing is a failure or a success. It just is. Whatever happens, we can learn, grow, and expand.

Vedic teachings remind us that everything changes *except* the infinite field of consciousness. Realizing this encourages us to enjoy the beautiful moments of life thoroughly while knowing they will change and not to worry too much when things are tough, because they, too, will pass. With this wisdom — which is a part of many traditions — we can engage in the world with a more grounded and secure mind.

The great yogi Sri Nisargadatta Maharaj said, "Consciousness is my home. It is love. It is who I truly am." When we are anchored in the love, spaciousness, and pure potential that is our essence, we don't hesitate to try new things. We've all heard spiritual teachers say we have boundless potential. How do we know if we don't explore it? This doesn't mean we won't fall many times in our pursuits. This doesn't mean we won't have to acquire new skills in a given subject. Whether you experience your full potential is not necessarily dependent on the outer world — on what opportunities the world gives you. It depends on you. How open are you to creating a life that honors your svadharma, even if you stumble along the way? How willing are you to do the legwork — the research, the study, the asking for help? How open are you to making choices in your life that help instead of harm you, that cultivate energy instead of drain it? How receptive are you to actively shaping your life instead of passively receiving it?

Remember how important your stories about yourself are. What is the story that you burned in Week Five? What is the new story that you have been cultivating? How do you remember it? By celebrating it. Have a dinner party. Invite your closest friends. Tell them about your new story. Rejoice together. It doesn't mean you won't struggle as you emerge into your new story. If you're like everyone I know, it is pretty much a given that you will face many challenges as you create a life of meaning and purpose that is aligned with your true potential and gifts. Don't hesitate to celebrate just because you know you will fall along the way. Celebrate because you *will* fall, and you *are* scared, but you are going for it anyway. Celebrate your courage and strength. Be a living inspiration for your friends, community, and children. Remember, children learn from what they see us do, not from what we tell them to do. Our words are nothing compared to our actions, which are a result of our thoughts — specifically, how we think about ourselves, our worth and capacity.

Celebration

Indian spirituality encompasses profound insights into behavioral sciences. Through Ayurveda and yoga, our behaviors become pleasant and harmonious. Adopt a healthy lifestyle, create a warm atmosphere, and make life a celebration.

SRI SRI RAVI SHANKAR

The fourth foundation of the Yogi's Way is nourishment. Immerse yourself in breath, movement, awareness, rest, and community. Cultivate a healthy lifestyle and make life a celebration. My greatest teacher on how to celebrate life was my grandmother, whose story I introduced in Week Five.

My grandmother taught me that a resilient and peaceful mind and living a meaningful and joyful life are possible no matter our outer circumstances. She was born in 1929 in Khandwa, a small town in Madhya Pradesh located in Central India. This was a time in India when it was normal for girls as young as fourteen to get married. It was also a time when India was under British colonial rule.

My grandmother's life wasn't easy. She was taken out of school in the eighth grade, at the age of fourteen, to marry my grandfather, a man she had never met, seen, or spoken with. She was a child. He was seven years her senior.

Upon marriage, my grandmother moved to Delhi with my grandfather, which was approximately a fifteen-hour train ride away from her home. She had no family or friends in Delhi. Pregnant for the first time at sixteen, she ended up having four daughters during a time in India when boys were preferred and women were looked down upon for not having at least one son. Still, my grandmother would proclaim, "I wish I had seven daughters!"

While my grandfather worked and lived abroad, my grand-mother raised her daughters on her own in Delhi. When she felt sad and alone, she allowed those emotions to come and go without letting them define or defeat her. Her life was full of hardship, taking care of a household and four young girls completely by herself in an extremely patriarchal society. In those days, it wasn't normal for a woman to be seen outside the home without being accompanied by a male figure, such as a husband, father, or brother. Yet my grandmother loved going out to run errands on her own, buying fresh vegetables every day from the vendors in the neighborhood and taking her girls to the parks and movies. My mother and her sisters always recall with astonishment how much joy she carried in her daily life.

My grandmother made friends in Delhi and cultivated a community. With them, she celebrated the festivals. She danced, sang, and lived with reverence. She sang mantra every morning and throughout the day. While cooking, cleaning, sewing, and running errands, she always had mantras moving through her mind. She was connected to her strength, love, intelligence, and creative energies within and around her. She sewed all her daughters' dresses, made every meal for them from scratch, and gave them constant love and tenderness. She fostered strong bonds with her friends, regularly inviting them to her home, where they would knit, crochet, and prepare pickles and snacks together, all while exchanging stories and updates about their lives.

A true warrior, my grandmother was amazing in how she overcame her kleshas. It's not that she didn't feel sad, lonely, overwhelmed, angry, and hurt at times. She did. But she knew her thoughts and emotions were temporary, belonging to the dimension where everything changes. She knew, "This, too, shall pass." She didn't let kleshas drain her energy or block her love for her daughters, her life, and herself. She allowed her emotions to come and go while remaining rooted in consciousness, our primal source of love, energy, healing, and possibility. Possibility doesn't necessarily mean traveling the world and doing a million different things. It can mean making your current circumstances beautiful and meaningful. My grandmother lived a joyful and purposeful life fueled by mantras, community, her daughters, and the unshakable love that she cultivated through them. She was able to forgive those who caused her the greatest pain.

In our youth, my cousin Sonia and I had many conversations with our grandmother, whom we called Granny. It was clear to us that Granny felt her pain when it was present. She just didn't grasp it, so there was always space within her to experience the juicy, sweet parts of day-to-day life as they were happening. She recognized the beautiful moments and rejoiced in them. Whether in the kitchen cooking one of her amazing meals or out running errands, Granny always moved in a way that was grounded and graceful. Never in a rush, she let her higher mind prevail. All of this enabled her to connect with the fifth layer of her body: the bliss body, described in Week Three. As you'll recall, beyond the physical, energetic, and mental layers of the body lies a sea of peace and joy. The Chandogya Upanishad (4.3) teaches that *only those who have purified the mind can find this world. This world is theirs alone. In this world, in all worlds, they live in perfect freedom.*

I remember visiting Granny in the hospital on one of her visits to the US. She was as relaxed sitting in a wheelchair about to go into heart surgery as she was reading a magazine on her couch at home. She carried a peace within her that was unshakable.

My mom shares a story of being at the airport with Granny. As they collected their bags to check in for an international flight, Mom suddenly realized she couldn't find Granny's passport. In a panic, Mom frantically searched their belongings. It took her about twenty minutes to find the passport. What was striking to my mom about this incident was how Granny didn't get shaken for a moment. Her body, voice, and expressions remained calm the entire time.

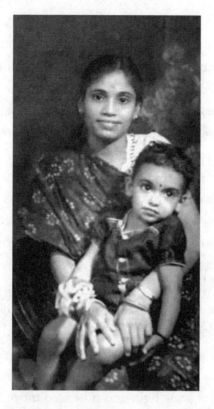

FIGURE 16: Granny holding my mother.

My family has countless stories like this about Granny. Jesus said he was in this world but not of it (John 17:16). Granny was in touch with a dimension that is available to all of us: consciousness, light, grace, possibility, a peace that passeth all understanding.

To live in perfect freedom is to live in the seat of consciousness — to let yourself be who you are in your soul and your spirit. At a soul level, we are the same: beings of infinite light and potential. On a spirit level, we carry a uniqueness that we long to experience and express. My grandmother expressed who she truly was in her soul and her spirit through her home, food, knitting, embroidery, friendships, motherhood, and resilience.

My grandmother was a living example that WE ARE capable

beyond measure and WE CAN live freely and fully despite the challenges life brings us. Granny's svadharma was to raise her daughters in a loving and joyful household, even if it had to be without her husband by her side for months, years, and decades. She did it, not always with ease and fearlessness, but with courage and faith in the light that lives inside her and all beings. My grandmother embodied the wisdom and essence of yoga.

The reason we adore our teachers in yoga lineages is because they show us what's possible. They are our mirrors, a living example of our own capacity. In this tradition, when we bow to our teacher, we bow to our potential. We water the seeds within us that they have cultivated within themselves. As we witness our teachers, spend time with them, acknowledge their generosity, patience, stability, wisdom, and love, we remember that these qualities live within us as well. The peace of my grandmother, the wisdom of my grandfather, the strength of my asana teacher, the serenity of my father, and the bliss of my mother and aunties who sing mantra reside within me too. The same light and potential move through us all. A true teacher is priceless, because what they give us is invaluable — vision, hope, and belief in ourselves.

My grandmother celebrated life by spending time with her daughters, friends, and community. She loved participating in *garba* and *raas*, folk dances that celebrate the many aspects of the Goddess. She enjoyed singing mantra by herself and with her community, playing cards with her grandchildren, picking flowers from the garden, and preparing delicious and nutritious homemade meals for her family.

Before reading further, reflect on the question, How do you celebrate life?

I used to associate celebrations with treats that involve lots of sugar and chocolate. Every time I wanted to rejoice for something good that happened in life, I would buy myself and my family and friends nice, sugary treats. Then, I started to change my thoughts. Why not celebrate life in ways that nurture us for the long term instead of providing temporary satiation?

Inspired by my grandmother, I have begun to celebrate life by spending time with loved ones, whether that is cooking a meal from scratch and inviting my best friends over for dinner, planning a weekend getaway with friends or family, or bringing a group together to share poetry, music, or a yoga practice. Community is the key. Together, we are better, stronger, and more resilient. We were born to lift each other up and celebrate life, even and especially amid hardship.

Week Twelve Practices

1. Bedtime Visualization:
Celebrate the Highest Version of Yourself

This week, every night as you lie in bed and close your eyes to fall asleep, take a few minutes to visualize the highest version of yourself. Refer to step 8 in the Week Eleven Meditation Prep (page 227). See your life as a blank canvas and paint a picture of yourself actualizing your deepest desires. Add as much detail as you can.

We are all artists. Make your life a masterpiece.

DANNY PARADISE

Allow yourself to experience the sensation of this vision being a reality. How does it feel to live up to your full potential? Tune in to your body, your heart, and your mind. Take your time to fully explore and immerse yourself in these sensations.

Express gratitude as though your vision has already manifested. In your own words, silently convey something like, *Thank you for bringing my dreams to fruition.* This act is immensely powerful. Fill your heart with gratitude as if your vision is now a reality.

2. Direct Your Energy

On this twelve-week journey we have learned to guard our gates and protect our energy from the people and things that unnecessarily drain us. Now, consider where you would like to place more of your energy. Is there a friend, family member, teacher, or community that you would like to connect with?

Remember the phenomenon of mirror neurons introduced in Week Seven. We tend to mirror the actions, habits, words, and characteristics of the people we surround ourselves with. Continue to apply this insight to your life now. In your journal, make a list of people who inspire you and who embody qualities that you would like to cultivate within yourself. Next to each of their names, write down the characteristics that you adore about them: perhaps discipline, passion, perseverance, humor, patience, courage, strength, warmth, kindness, sincerity. Would you want to place a picture of them, a quote by them, or an image that reminds you of them in your practice space? The outer and inner worlds reflect each other. Keep nurturing your practice space and your mind.

The dedicated children's rights activist Marian Wright Edelman said, "You can't be what you can't see." This is precisely why in yoga traditions we surround ourselves with inspiration, whether that be a community, a teacher, a mitra, or images of inspiring beings. Where we direct our energy and what and whom we choose to surround ourselves with profoundly shape our thoughts and lives.

In Week Ten, we began to look at our svadharma and ask ourselves what we are drawn to. Check in with yourself again. Is there a skill you would like to learn or refine, a course you feel inclined to take, something new you would like to explore? Is there a direction in which your spirit wants to expand? Listen and journal about what arises. Allow your spirit to communicate freely, even if the words are clumsy. Embrace the flow of expression.

3. Rejoice

Celebration is a universal tradition, deeply rooted in collective history. Throughout the world, people come together to celebrate significant events such as festivals, holidays, achievements, and rites of passages. These celebrations often involve storytelling, music, dance, and feasting, all of which foster a sense of community and continuity. The act of celebrating, whether simple or grand, is a powerful way to acknowledge and share the joys of life and reinforce connections that unite us as humans.

Recognizing and celebrating successes, both big and small, plays a crucial role in sustaining motivation, reinforcing positive habits, and enhancing a sense of fulfillment. Research indicates that recognizing even small achievements activates the brain's reward pathways, releasing dopamine, which boosts self-worth, confidence, motivation, and personal competence. Conversely, neglecting to celebrate can lead to chronic stress, burnout, and decreased motivation. Marking milestones helps us reinforce lessons learned and deepen our connection with others, making celebration key to personal and professional growth.

Setting clear goals lays the foundation for acknowledging your wins, no matter the size. Additionally, deciding in advance how you will celebrate small and big milestones boosts your motivation and makes it more likely that you will indeed take the time to celebrate when the moment arrives.

Celebration doesn't need to wait for a particular achievement. It can be as simple as honoring and sharing the joy of being alive. Compile a list of five to ten ways to infuse your life with celebration. For example, you might write:

- I will start a gratitude journal.
- I will go on a daily walk and enjoy the fresh air.
- I will reach out to my closest friends and start planning our fiftieth birthday bash.
- I will invite my neighbor to enjoy Sun Salutations with me once a week.
- I will make a coffee date with a friend so we can discuss and celebrate each other's latest wins.

These actions may seem small, but they will carry a powerful impact.

4. Share the Love

Spirituality and service go hand in hand.
Yoga makes us perfectly fit and socially useful.

My grandfather NARENDRA KUMAR

How do you master something? By teaching it. Research in the learning sciences reveals the truth of a proverb attributed to the Roman philosopher Seneca the Younger two thousand years ago: "By teaching, we learn." The best way to integrate something is to explain it to someone else. When you teach, you cultivate a solid understanding of a subject. You also realize gaps in your knowledge, recognize mistakes, and make improvements. Teaching requires you to repeat things again and again, making it more likely you'll retain what you've learned and establish new habits. Teaching also makes you accountable to others. You are more inclined to maintain your practices in order to avoid an embarrassment or loss of credibility in front of another. When you teach, you are also more likely to stay inspired to practice.

Think of a friend, colleague, or family member who you feel would benefit from and appreciate learning any of the practices in this book. As an act of service, offer to be this person's mitra and share at least one of the practices with them. Perhaps it is the fire puja, Sun Salutations, KTL, ADY, or Guard Your Gates practice. Reflect on what you would like to share and with whom. Be a blessing to this person. As you share with them, you will integrate those teachings more deeply into your being and prepare yourself for further study. You might even consider going through the entire book with someone who you feel would gain from this twelve-week journey. Take a moment to jot down in your journal the names of those you might want to share some or all of this journey with.

I slept and dreamt that life was joy. I awoke and saw that life was service. I acted and behold, service was joy.

RABINDRANATH TAGORE

If you are free, you need to free somebody else. If you have some power, then your job is to empower somebody else.

TONI MORRISON

5. Enjoy Your Daily Practice

Celebrate how far you have come! Often celebration is accompanied with gifts. The gift you have cultivated for yourself is a personal yoga practice that is healing and holistic. This week, enjoy bringing together the powerful practices you have learned on this twelve-week journey.

Below is a suggested way to integrate everything you've learned, dividing the exercises into a morning and an evening session. If you prefer to do them all in one session, that's perfectly fine. This is for you to do at your own rhythm and in your own time. Experiment with what works best in your life. Know that however you choose to practice, your mitras, friends, family, and community are celebrating your journey with you.

As you practice to embody the highest version of yourself and live your life with integrity, you create an energy that affects all beings. Through your determination, courage, and strength, you may inspire someone or many people on the other side of the world whom you've never even met, because you are bringing an empowering and liberating vibration to the whole of life. Remember, when you bring forth what is within you, it doesn't have to be fancy. A genuine smile, a kind word, or an embrace can be the most potent gift that a moment calls for.

The Yogi's Way Heal Yourself Now®
Seventy-Minute Sequence

Morning Practice

1. In My Own Hands practice: fifteen seconds
2. Optimal Breath practice: three minutes (ideally, add Meditation Prep here: three minutes, totaling six minutes)
3. All-Day Yoga
4. Sun Salutations with mantras and chakra awareness: fifteen to twenty minutes
5. Witness Meditation followed by Consciousness Meditation: six minutes each
6. Savasana: five minutes
7. Journaling: five minutes (reflecting on the above practices)

Total morning practice time: approximately forty-five minutes

Evening Practice

1. Ayurveda Awareness Journal: three minutes
2. Alternate between Klesha Trigger Log and Check Your Heart, Change Your Thoughts practices on one day and Free Journaling the next: fifteen to twenty minutes
3. Bedtime visualization: five minutes

Total evening practice time: approximately twenty-five minutes

Week Twelve Mitra Meeting

Go over the last twelve weeks with your mitras and discuss which practices and teachings moved you the most and which you are most excited to continue. (See appendix A on page 261 for a review of the main practices from the last twelve weeks.) What are the ways you are choosing to celebrate life? Whom are you inclined to share some or all of the practices in this book with? Plan a date with your mitras a month from now to celebrate one another for completing this twelve-week journey.

CONCLUSION

Peace Is Possible

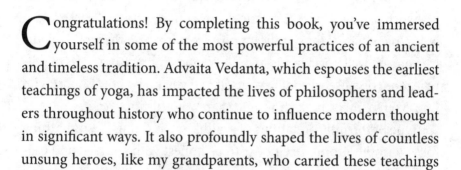

Congratulations! By completing this book, you've immersed yourself in some of the most powerful practices of an ancient and timeless tradition. Advaita Vedanta, which espouses the earliest teachings of yoga, has impacted the lives of philosophers and leaders throughout history who continue to influence modern thought in significant ways. It also profoundly shaped the lives of countless unsung heroes, like my grandparents, who carried these teachings deep in their souls, allowing love and understanding to permeate every aspect of their lives and touch everyone they encountered.

According to Vedic tradition, one of the primary purposes of spiritual practice is experiencing *moksha*, which translates as "freedom," "liberation," or "release." It signifies the transformative realization that the individual soul shares the same boundless light and potential as ultimate reality. Through life's highs and lows, this light remains untainted. Vedic philosophers' views align with those of today's quantum physicists, who assert that the fundamental nature of both individuals and the universe is pure potentiality.

Our connection to this quantum dimension depends on our state of mind. A mind clouded by kleshas blocks us from exploring the infinite field of possibility, which in this tradition is called "consciousness." This is why liberating the mind from harmful tendencies is pivotal on the yogic path.

Over the past twelve weeks, you've committed to numerous powerful practices, all geared toward fostering a direct connection with consciousness and unlocking the door to ultimate freedom. With sustained practice and integration, the mind can emerge as a healing force, refreshing your inner landscape and the world around you. Get ready to experience the transformative ripple effect in your relationships and life. As you evolve, peace becomes more of a possibility — one thought and one choice at a time.

At this juncture of your journey, if you're unsure about your svadharma, don't worry. Just know that you possess a purpose and it holds the potential for significant positive impact on the world. Nourish yourself well, revel in the joys of life, and embrace practices of self-reflection, because you value yourself and you know how important it is for you to uncover, nurture, and share your distinctive gifts.

One of the interpretations of svadharma is doing the right thing for you in *this* moment. Choose to be honest with yourself and others in each moment, and your purpose will reveal itself. Doors will open. Often, it is essential to slow down and remove all that is unnecessary in our lives to notice the possibilities that emerge when we begin honoring our deepest desires.

A Chinese proverb states: "There are many paths to the top of the mountain, but the view is always the same." The view is of love, unity, and possibility. What I've offered in this book isn't the only way to practice yoga by any means. It is one way to honor yoga's roots, which lie in the mind and consciousness.

As the world changes in ways that are making us more isolated, it is essential to gather mitras on our journey. This way, no matter what arises as we engage in our inner practices, we have the support of friends. Doing this work alone can cause stress and anxiety. With our mitras, however, we can pick up the phone when needed and know that they will be there for us, listening with that same open, welcoming consciousness that we are learning to live in.

Motivation is also important to establish early on the path. If our motivation is to create peace and healing only for ourselves, we may falter on our journey. Cultivating the wish to contribute our gifts and be a benefit to others is powerful. Understanding how our thoughts and emotions affect our health is also foundational, because it inspires us to work through destructive patterns and cultivate nurturing ones. Realizing that we have a choice in every moment about what we think, say, and do is essential. Writing our story in such a way as to claim our power creates the foundation for merging with our true potential.

As we engage in yoga practices, it is of paramount importance to ground ourselves in the affectionate and loving seat of consciousness, because our practices often open us to our wounds. Love allows us to accept and be with our pain and with the full spectrum of human emotions. Such presence creates space for us to connect with the wisdom that underlies emotion and eventually to free ourselves of the grip that kleshas often have on us.

In this book, you've been introduced to the four foundations of the Yogi's Way: motivation, stories, choices, and nourishment. You've also learned about the twelve pillars: mitras, breath, healthy thoughts, mantra, visualization, meditation, movement, rest, journaling, communication, nutrition, and service. Each of these foundations and pillars is explored in more depth in subsequent in-person and online programs of the Yogi's Way (see "Next Steps" page 259).

Ultimately, yoga awakens us to our creative potential. In Sanskrit, the latent energies we stir through yoga practices are called *shakti*. Shakti is an inner wellspring of fresh, vibrant, innovative energy. As we practice, our innate power surfaces, and we summon the courage to follow its call.

When I was in my midtwenties, my mother shared this valuable lesson with me: "Always surround yourself with individuals who have greater knowledge and experience than you." If it wasn't for her wisdom, I might not have found myself working alongside a world-renowned oncologist in New York City or meditating with shamans in the Brazilian Amazon. As your creative energy rises, be receptive to the many teachers and teachings that surround you. Stay humble, open, and present. It is our nature to expand. The learning doesn't end. We never reach our full potential, because it is infinite. We're always students of life. Echoing my mother's insight, may you always place yourself in a position to learn and grow, because it is your nature to do so.

Most importantly, enjoy your journey. Make life a celebration. Embrace the beauty of having goals for healing, growth, and expansion. Equally, cherish the present moment and cultivate gratitude. The more we appreciate life, the greater our joy. Even this phenomenon is being discovered by science.

Begin and end each day by giving thanks for the miracle of being alive and having a soul and a world that offer boundless possibilities.

Concluding Practice: Love Who You Are

Remember the summit of wisdom we explored in Week Eight? Spiritual traditions worldwide remind us that we are all divine beings, each carrying the same light as our essence. Amid humanity's rich diversity, we share this fundamental unity.

Vedic texts teach us that if you see the Divine as separate from yourself, you have not yet understood ultimate truth. Tat Tvam Asi — "You are that." You are inseparable from the highest reality: boundless light and possibility. This is a reality that does not change. Individuals such as entrepreneur Madam C. J. Walker and Holocaust survivors Dr. Edith Eva Eger and Dr. Viktor Frankl show us that this truth endures, even in the face of the most oppressive life circumstances. You carry the same infinite potential as the people you admire most in this world, though your gifts are unique. As introduced in Week Eight, an indigenous song in South America expresses, "The medicine that cures me is the medicine that cures everyone: We are all God."

In closing, I offer you one more simple but powerful practice. The purpose of the Love Who You Are practice below is to help you remember your essence and love yourself wherever you are on your journey. You don't have to wait to achieve anything to honor yourself now. You are alive, breathing, and abounding with possibility now.

This practice helps to develop a mindset where, when you look in the mirror, you can say without hesitation, "I love you." It doesn't require you to take any extra time out of your day.

Love Who You Are

- When you wake up in the morning, as you brush your teeth and look in the mirror, say to yourself, "I am brushing the teeth of a divine being."
- When you shower or bathe, say to yourself, "I am washing the body of a divine being."
- When you come out of the bath, say to yourself, "I am dressing the body of a divine being." Then, "I am combing the hair of a divine being."
- As you make yourself your morning drink and breakfast, say to yourself, "I am nourishing the body of a divine being."
- Before you start your activities for the rest of your day — be they caring for your children, going out to work, or working on a project at home — take one last look in the mirror. Whether you are feeling tired or fresh, old or young, anxious or relaxed, see the face of the Divine — infinite love and possibility. Remember you are not your changing body, thoughts, or emotions. You are the Self that can guide the mind and body with wisdom and love. You are light. Inhale

slowly into the center of your heart. Exhale and say, internally or out loud, "I love you."

When you engage in this practice, feel free to replace "a divine being" with "a precious being," "a sacred being," "a goddess," or any other term that resonates with you.

This path gives you a beautiful balance of confidence and humility. We cultivate the confidence to know that we are precious and divine while recognizing that *everyone* carries the same essence.

In 2016, I taught the Yogi's Way Love Who You Are practice to a group of teacher trainees. One of the students, Marisa, shared with our community that after a few weeks of doing this practice (she used the term "goddess" to address herself), her husband began treating her differently. One Saturday morning, he brought her breakfast in bed, something he had never done in their twenty-five years of marriage. He started buying her flowers, another new act of love. She was astonished. She hadn't told him about the practice. But when she saw herself as a goddess, worthy of love, these miraculous things happened.

Another student, Janet, shared that this practice helped her to finally, at the age of thirty-five, genuinely experience self-love and self-worth. The miracle for Janet was that she felt this love, not because of how others treated her, but because of how she began to see and treat herself.

As we begin to view ourselves as divine beings, we can see others in the same light. For example, we may begin to view our spouse, children, colleagues, or even a perfect stranger as divine. This shift in perception inspires positive changes in how we relate to ourselves and others.* One day, an eternal truth preserved in the Vedas may

---

*   One caution: If you are in an abusive situation, don't convince yourself to stay because your abuser's essence is divine. Leave. Be safe. From afar, hold that person in light and pray for their healing.

resonate within our own being: Vasudhaiva Kutumbakam — "The world is one family."

By becoming practitioners of yoga, we dismantle patterns within that harm ourselves and others, while cultivating ones that nurture an enduring peace for all.

Next Steps

We have covered a lot of ground in this book. You may want to go right back to the beginning and experience it all again. If so, go for it. As you now know, repetition is powerful.

The teachings and practices in this book provide a strong foundation while paving the way for deeper exploration. TheYogisWay .com offers additional online and in-person programs to further enhance your practice. For instance, the pranic winds and energy centers introduced in Week Three have profound implications for our practice and health, which are explored more fully in later programs. Additionally, there are many more mantras to learn and experience, each offering unique support on your journey.

If you struggle with a particular klesha, the Yogi's Way offers Yoga for Emotional Resilience, a series of eight courses featuring specific yoga sequences to help you navigate each of the major kleshas introduced in this book. Each course includes its own sadhana — a dedicated set of practices incorporating movement, breathing exercises, mantra, visualization, and subtle body awareness, as well as wisdom teachings and contemplations to address that specific klesha. The movement components of these programs include circular and spiral motions, inspired by Indian classical dance and personal insight.

With a solid foundation and further studies of the subtle body, we ultimately design personalized yoga sequences to help practitioners move through kleshas. The Yogi's Way tailors these sequences to meet the specific physical, emotional, mental, and spiritual needs of each practitioner. For example, for female practitioners, topics related to fertility, pregnancy, postpartum care, menopause, and hormonal changes are addressed when relevant.

For those interested in teacher training, this book constitutes Module 1 of the Yogi's Way 500-hour program. Information for online and in-person teacher trainings is available at TheYogisWay.com.

BUILDING *THE YOGI'S WAY* HEAL YOURSELF NOW® SEQUENCE

A Healing and Holistic Practice

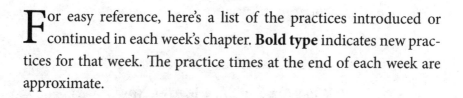

For easy reference, here's a list of the practices introduced or continued in each week's chapter. **Bold type** indicates new practices for that week. The practice times at the end of each week are approximate.

Week One: Mitras

Choose Your Mitras
Find Your Motivation
Journey Inward
Establish Boundaries
Seek Blessings

Week Two: Kleshas

Recognize Your Kleshas
Klesha Trigger Log
Five-Minute Optimal Breath Practice
All-Day Yoga

Total daily practice time: ten to fifteen minutes

Week Three: Subtle Body, Physical Body

Subtle Body Awareness
Ujjayi Pranayama
Five-minute Optimal Breath practice
All-Day Yoga
Fifteen-minute Sun Salutations with chakra awareness
Five-minute Savasana
Journaling
Klesha Trigger Log

Total daily practice time: thirty-five to forty-five minutes

Week Four: Consciousness

WAYEN: What Are You Experiencing Now?
Three-minute Optimal Breath practice (**add: connect with the heart, invite positive emotions**)
All-Day Yoga
Fifteen-minute Sun Salutations with chakra awareness
Six-minute Witness Meditation
Five-minute Savasana
Journaling
Klesha Trigger Log

Total daily practice time: forty to fifty minutes

Week Five: Stories

Write down three mantras daily
Release Your Labels
Examine Your Story
Fire ceremony
Fifteen-second In My Own Hands practice

Three-minute Optimal Breath practice
All-Day Yoga (**add: optional So ham mantra**)
Fifteen-minute Sun Salutations with chakra awareness
Six-minute Witness Meditation
Five-minute Space Meditation
Five-minute Savasana
Journaling
Klesha Trigger Log

Total daily practice time: forty-five to fifty-five minutes

Week Six: Mantra

Fifteen-second In My Own Hands practice
Three-minute Optimal Breath practice
All-Day Yoga (add: optional So ham mantra)
**Ten-minute daily review of twelve Sun Salutation
mantras**
Fifteen-minute Sun Salutations with chakra awareness
Six-minute Witness Meditation
Five-minute Savasana
Journaling
Klesha Trigger Log

Total daily practice time: fifty to sixty minutes

Week Seven: Choices

Guard Your Gates practice (variable timing)
Fifteen-second In My Own Hands practice
Three-minute Optimal Breath practice
All-Day Yoga
Ten-minute daily review of twelve Sun Salutation man-
tras

Fifteen-minute Sun Salutations with chakra awareness
Six-minute Witness Meditation
Five-minute Savasana
Journaling
Klesha Trigger Log

Total daily practice time: fifty to sixty minutes (plus Guard Your Gates practice time)

Week Eight: The Summit of Wisdom

Contemplate the klesha of delusion
Fifteen-second In My Own Hands practice
Three-minute Optimal Breath practice
All-Day Yoga
Fifteen- to twenty-minute Sun Salutations with chakra
    awareness **and mantras**
Six-minute Witness Meditation
Five-minute Savasana
Journaling
Klesha Trigger Log
Weekly Joy Practice

Total daily practice time: forty to fifty-five minutes

Week Nine: Alchemy

**Check Your Heart, Change Your Thoughts journaling
    practice**
Fifteen-second In My Own Hands practice
Three-minute Optimal Breath practice
All-Day Yoga
Fifteen- to twenty-minute Sun Salutations with chakra
    awareness and mantras

Six-minute Witness Meditation
Five-minute Savasana
Journaling
Klesha Trigger Log
Weekly Joy Practice

Total daily practice time: fifty to sixty minutes

Week Ten: Self-Healing

Ayurvedic Constitution questionnaire
Ayurvedic Guidelines for Healthful Eating
Explore your Svadharma
Fifteen-second In My Own Hands practice
Three-minute Optimal Breath practice
All-Day Yoga
Fifteen- to twenty-minute Sun Salutation with chakra
    awareness and mantras
Six-minute Witness Meditation
Five-minute Savasana
Three-minute Ayurveda Awareness Journal
Klesha Trigger Log or Check Your Heart, Change Your
    Thoughts
Free Journaling
Weekly Joy Practice

Total daily practice time: fifty to sixty minutes

Week Eleven: Meditation

Fifteen-second In My Own Hands practice
Three-minute Meditation Prep
Three-minute Optimal Breath practice (can be part of
    Meditation Prep, making the Meditation Prep ap-
    proximately six minutes

All-Day Yoga

Fifteen- to twenty-minute Sun Salutation with chakra
    awareness and mantras

Six-minute Witness Meditation

Six-minute Consciousness Meditation

Five-minute Savasana

Three-minute Ayurveda Awareness Journal

Klesha Trigger Log or Check Your Heart, Change Your
    Thoughts

Journaling

Weekly Joy Practice

Total daily practice time: sixty to seventy minutes

Week Twelve: Service and Celebration

Five-minute Bedtime Visualization
Daily Celebrations of Life list
Service to a New Mitra
The Yogi's Way seventy-minute Heal Yourself Now®
sequence

Total daily practice time: seventy minutes, as described on page 250.

THE SUN SALUTATION PRACTICE WITH MANTRA AND CHAKRA AWARENESS

In this course, we delved into a potent practice called Surya Na-maskara, or Sun Salutations. In Week Three, we learned the twelve movements of this sequence, along with understanding the chakra, or energy center, activated by each pose. In Week Six, we learned the twelve accompanying mantras, or affirmations, and dedicated two weeks to contemplating their significance. While expressing gratitude for the qualities of light the mantras represent, we acknowledged their presence within us.

In Week Eight, we further deepened our practice by reciting one mantra at the beginning of each round of the twelve-step Sun Salutation sequence. Beginning with the first mantra in Mountain Pose, we contemplated its essence throughout the sequence's twelve postures. This method, repeated for six to twelve rounds, is a personal favorite.

Alternatively, you may recite one mantra with every individual movement within the twelve-step practice, repeating this cycle up to twelve times. A visual representation of both approaches is available at TheYogisWay.com/thebook. For those interested in exploring the second method, a concise summary is provided below.

As we integrate breath, movement, and mantra, we ultimately embody the radiant qualities of the sun, becoming a light to ourselves and others.

What your mind dwells on you become.

Brihadaranyaka Upanishad

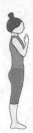

1. Om Mitraya Namah: "Friendly and affectionate to all." *Heart chakra: acceptance, compassion, to love and be loved.*

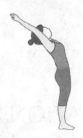

2. Om Ravaye Namah: "Cause for change." *Throat chakra: to speak and be heard.*

3. Om Suryaye Namah: "Inspires action." *Sacral chakra: to feel and to want.*

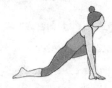

4. Om Bhanave Namah: "Diffuses light." *Third eye chakra: to see, imagine, intuit.*

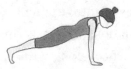

5. Om Khagaye Namah: "Moves through obstacles." *Throat chakra: to speak and be heard.*

6. Om Pushne Namah: "Nourishes all." *Solar plexus chakra: to act with confidence and will.*

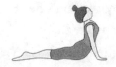

7. Om Hiranyagarbhaya Namah: "Brings healing." *Sacral chakra: to feel and to want.*

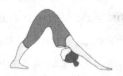

8. Om Marichaye Namah: "Illumines truth." *Throat chakra: to speak and be heard.*

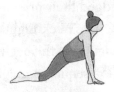

9. Om Adityaya Namah: "Respect to the cosmic mother, whose light lives within all." *Third eye chakra: to see, imagine, intuit.*

10. Om Savitre Namah: "Creates everything." *Sacral chakra: to feel and to want.*

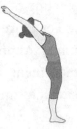

11. Om Arkaya Namah: "Removes afflictions, is worthy of praise." *Throat chakra: to speak and be heard.*

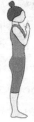

12. Om Arkaya Namah: "Illumines wisdom." *Heart chakra: acceptance, compassion, to love and be loved.*

ACKNOWLEDGMENTS

I extend my deepest gratitude to my family of teachers, especially my grandparents, mother, and father. They imparted the wisdom of ancient Vedic texts and exemplified the transformative essence of yoga through their resilience and courage. To my daughter, Mila: your radiant presence fueled me through the entire journey of writing this book. Thank you for all the evenings you sat by my side reading those big volumes of *Harry Potter* as I wrote these pages.

Thank you for your teachings, Sri Nisargadatta Maharaj, Sri Ramana Maharshi, Paramahansa Yogananda, Anandamayi Ma, Venerable Thupten Phuntsok, Douglas Veenhof, Larry Schultz, Danny Paradise, and Ma Daya Vyas.

Thank you to my cherished circle of friends, my mitras, who supported me with unwavering encouragement as well as feedback on multiple drafts of this work: Sonia Shah, Lynn Gray, Della Dumlao, Angie Prewitt, Susan Zafer, Mike Murphy, Molly Dahl, and Tad Fettig. Your time, care, and friendship are invaluable and precious to me. Thank you, Mitch Hall, my editorial consultant, for sharing the depth of your care, wisdom, and skills.

Thank you, George Greenfield, my literary and speaking agent, for your gracious and steadfast support. Your belief in me has been instrumental in bringing this book to life. My heartfelt appreciation to my publisher and editor, Georgia Hughes, as well as Diana Rico, Kristen Cashman, Tracy Cunningham, Tona Pearce Myers, Kim Corbin, and the rest of the wonderful team at New World Library. It's an honor to be a part of your literary family.

Thank you to my brother and sister-in-law, Vishal and Shetal Datta, and extended family for being a treasured part of my life. And thank you to my students, for your courage in exploring the depths of the mind and heart and for cultivating the discipline and patience to make lasting change. There are so many people I adore who have blessed my path and made this book possible. With all my heart, thank you.

NOTES

Introduction

p. 2 *Love, forgiveness, hope, and connection*: Bruce H. Lipton, *The Biology of Belief: Unleashing the Power of Consciousness, Matter, and Miracles* (Hay House, 2005).

p. 2 *Research consistently reveals*: Lakshmi Menezes, "What Is the Mind-Body Connection?," Florida Medical Clinic, August 24, 2020, https://www.floridamedicalclinic.com/blog/what-is-the-mind-body-connection/.

p. 3 *It's been estimated that 72 percent*: Ryan Peacock, "7 Things I Learned about Women from Doing Yoga," *Yoga Journal*, September 2, 2021, https://www.yogajournal.com/lifestyle/7-things-i-learned-about-women-from-doing-yoga/#.

p. 3 *Women consistently make up*: Anna Fleck, "Who's Practicing Yoga?," Statista, June 21, 2023, https://www.statista.com/chart/27653/yoga-men-and-women-by-country/.

p. 7 *A spiritual warrior is someone*: In Eknath Easwaran's translations of the Bhagavad Gita, he expresses that an indomitable will, courage, and endurance are required on the path of yoga. *Bhagavad Gita for Daily Living Volume 2: Like a Thousand Suns* (Nilgiri Press, 1979), 27.

p. 9 *"Even a cursory glance of yoga scriptures"*: Narendra Kumar, *Introduction to Vedanta* (Manav Mandir Publications, 1992), 54.

p. 9 *"As different streams having their sources in different places"*: Rigveda 1.164, quoted in Kumar, *Introduction to Vedanta*, 55.

p. 10 *"a latent human capacity"*: Michael Murphy, *The Future of the Body: Explorations into the Further Evolution of Human Nature* (Jeremy P. Tarcher, 1992), 72.

Week One: Mitras

p. 17 *"Call it a clan, call it a network"*: Jane Howard, *Families* (1978; repr., Transaction Publishers, 1999), 234.

p. 18   *"epidemic of loneliness and isolation"*: Vivek Murthy, quoted in "New Surgeon General Advisory Raises Alarm about the Devastating Impact of the Epidemic of Loneliness and Isolation in the United States," US Department of Health and Human Services, May 3, 2023, https://www .hhs.gov/about/news/2023/05/03/new-surgeon-general-advisory-raises -alarm-about-devastating-impact-epidemic-loneliness-isolation-united -states.html.

p. 19   *"rebuilding social connection must be"*: Vivek Murthy, "The Loneliness Epidemic in America," *New York Times*, April 30, 2023, https://www .nytimes.com/2023/04/30/opinion/loneliness-epidemic-america.html.

p. 19   *Big tech has invested billions*: *The Social Dilemma*, directed by Jeff Orlowski-Yang (Exposure Labs, 2020).

p. 20   *The American Society of Training and Development*: Thomas Oppong, "Psychological Secrets to Hack Your Way to Better Life Habits," *Observer* (blog), March 20, 2017, https://observer.com/2017/03/psychological -secrets-hack-better-life-habits-psychology-productivity/.

p. 20   *about 54 percent of people*: Oppong, "Psychological Secrets."

p. 21   *In her research on the science*: Sonja Lyubomirsky, in "Acts of Kindness Are the Key to Happiness: Study," CBC Documentaries, December 15, 2022, https://www.cbc.ca/documentaries/the-passionate-eye/acts-of -kindness-are-the-key-to-happiness-study-1.6682912.

p. 24   *"Yoga helps us minimize kleshas"*: Swami Satchidananda, trans., *The Yoga Sutras of Patanjali* (Integral Yoga Publications, 2001), 83.

p. 24   *"We conquer every struggle within"*: My translation, adapted from Eknath Easwaran, trans., *The Upanishads* (Nilgiri Press, 2007), 260.

p. 25   *"Desire the good"*: Sri Nisargadatta Maharaj, *I Am That*, trans. Maurice Frydman (Chetana, 1973), 57.

p. 25   *"Children don't do what we say"*: Dr. Edith Eva Eger, interview with Oprah Winfrey, "The Choice," episode of *Oprah's Super Soul* (podcast), June 23, 2019, https://podcasts.apple.com/us/podcast/dr-edith-eva-eger -the-choice/id1264843400?i=1000442517079.

p. 26   *"The need to please people"*: "When the Body Says No — Caring for Our- selves While Caring for Others: Dr. Gabor Maté" (lecture), YouTube video, 1:15:47, posted March 6, 2013, https://www.youtube.com/watch?v=c6IL 8WVyMMs.

p. 27   *"The automatic and compulsive concern"*: Maté, "When the Body Says No."

p. 28   *"If you don't know how to say"*: Maté, "When the Body Says No."

Week Two: Kleshas

p. 33   *"There is no greater victory"*: Swami Ramdas, quoted in Eknath Easwaran, *The End of Sorrow* (Nilgiri Press, 1979), 46.

p. 33   *"What's the bravest thing"*: Charlie Mackesy, *The Boy, the Mole, the Fox, and the Horse* (HarperOne, 2019).

p. 34   *"Behold the Kurus"*: Eknath Easwaran, trans., *The Bhagavad Gita* (Nigiri Press, 2007), 79. Easwaran's translation is: "Arjuna, behold all the Kurus gathered together" (1.25).

p. 36   *"In the morning I bathe my intellect"*: Henry David Thoreau, *Walden* (Crowell & Co., 1910), 393.

p. 37   *"Everybody wants to let go"*: Devi, quoted in Daniel Odier, *Tantric Quest* (Inner Traditions, 1997), 59.

p. 39   *"the intensely painful feeling"*: Brené Brown, "Shame vs. Guilt," Brené Brown (website), January 15, 2013, https://brenebrown.com/articles /2013/01/15/shame-v-guilt/.

p. 39   *Major depressive disorder is*: Anxiety and Depression Association of America, "Anxiety Disorders: Facts & Statistics," updated October 28, 2022, https://adaa.org/understanding-anxiety/facts-statistics.

p. 39   *over 37 million Americans*: Michael Hastings, "More Than 37 Million Americans Take Antidepressants, Authors Say," *Winston-Salem Journal*, March 12, 2020, https://journalnow.com/life-entertainment/home-garden /article_36f2f74b-e268-5731-bdc0-d92a036d2cd4.html.

p. 40   *affecting about 40 million adults*: Anxiety and Depression Association of America, "Anxiety Disorders: Facts & Statistics."

p. 40   *301 million people suffer*: World Health Organization, "Anxiety Disorders," September 27, 2023, https://www.who.int/news-room/fact-sheets /detail/anxiety-disorders#:~:text=An%20estimated%204%25%20of%20 the,all%20mental%20disorders%20(1).

p. 43   *"When you know better"*: Maya Angelou, quoted in Oprah Winfrey, *What I Know for Sure* (Flatiron Books, 2014), 191.

p. 44   *a 5.5-second inhalation*: James Nestor, *Breath: The New Science of a Lost Art* (Riverhead Books, 2020), 83, 104.

p. 45   *the average person takes*: Nestor, *Breath*, 5.

p. 45   *nearly 50 percent of people*: Nestor, *Breath*, 5.

Week Three: Subtle Body, Physical Body

p. 52   *"Everything you're thinking and feeling"*: "Dr. Mitch Gaynor: The Harmonic Destiny of Healing," YouTube video, 24:44, posted October 29, 2015, https://www.youtube.com/watch?v=TFps22bWFI4.

p. 54   *"Focused on the senses and body"*: Eknath Easwaran, *Essence of the Upanishads* (Nilgiri Press, 2009), 65.

p. 55   *breakdown of the five winds*: Sandra Anderson, "The 5 Prana Vayus in Yoga," *Yoga International*, https://yogainternational.com/article/view/the-5-prana-vayus-in-yoga-prana; oral teachings at the Yoga Studies Institute, Tucson, Arizona, 2009–2010.

p. 57   *The flow of prana through*: S. Saraswati, *Surya Namaskara: A Technique of Solar Vitalization* (1983; repr., Yoga Publications Trust, 2015), 30–33; A. Judith, *Wheels of Life* (Llewellyn Publications, 1987), 3.

p. 59   *our thoughts, emotions, and beliefs profoundly influence*: D. Church, *Mind to Matter: The Astonishing Science of How Your Brain Creates Material Reality* (Hay House, 2018).

p. 60   *shame is linked to negative changes*: L. Dolezal and B. Lyons, "Health-Related Shame: An Affective Determinant of Health?," *Medical Humanities* 43, no. 4 (June 2017): 257–63, https://mh.bmj.com/content/43/4/257.

p. 60   *Loneliness significantly heightens*: Centers for Disease Control and Prevention, "Health Effects of Social Isolation and Loneliness," March 26, 2024, https://www.cdc.gov/social-connectedness/risk-factors/index.html.

p. 60   *Anger and anxiety disorders are associated*: C. M. Celano, D. J. Daunis, H. N. Lokko, K. A. Campbell, and J. C. Huffman, "Anxiety Disorders and Cardiovascular Disease," *Current Psychiatry Reports* 18 (September 26, 2016), https://doi.org/10.1007/s11920-016-0739-5.

p. 60   *Compassion is connected*: Steve Siegle, "The Art of Kindness," Mayo Clinic Health System, August 17, 2023, https://www.mayoclinic healthsystem.org/hometown-health/speaking-of-health/the-art-of-kindness.

p. 60   *Inner peace is associated with*: "The Benefits of Inner Peace," World Peace Initiative, https://wpifoundation.org/docs/ru/inner-peace-benefits#:~:text=It%2520increases%2520blood%2520flow%2520and,people%2520with%2520high%2520blood%2520pressure.

p. 60   *low self-worth can contribute*: J. F. Sowislo and U. Orth, "Does Low Self-Esteem Predict Depression and Anxiety? A Meta-analysis of Longitudinal Studies," *Psychological Bulletin* 139 (2013): 213–40, https://doi.org/10.1037/a0028931.

p. 60   *greater self-worth is linked*: H. Du, R. B. King, and P. Chi, "Self-Esteem and Subjective Well-Being Revisited: The Roles of Personal, Relational, and Collective Self-Esteem," *PLOS ONE* 12, no. 8 (August 25, 2017): e0183958, https://doi.org/10.1371/journal.pone.0183958.

p. 60   *Optimism is associated with*: L. O. Lee et al., "Optimism Is Associated with Exceptional Longevity in 2 Epidemiologic Cohorts of Men and Women," *Proceedings of the National Academy of Sciences* 116, no. 37 (September 10, 2019): 18357–62, https://doi.org/10.1073/pnas.1900712116.

p. 60   *A study on the placebo effect*: K. Meissner et al., "The Placebo Effect: Advances from Different Methodological Approaches," *The Journal of Neuroscience* 31, no. 45 (November 9, 2011): 16117–24, https://doi.org/10.1523/JNEUROSCI.4099-11.2011.

p. 60   *evidence suggesting that beliefs and emotions*: S. D. Pressman, B. N. Jenkins, and J. T. Moskowitz, "Positive Affect and Health: What Do We Know and Where Next Should We Go?," *Annual Review of Psychology* 70 (January 2019): 627–50, https://doi.org/10.1146/annurev-psych-010418-102955.

p. 62   *"I fear not the man who has practiced"*: Bruce Lee, quoted in Chelsea Cain, *One Kick*, reissue ed. (Pocket Books, 2015).

p. 64   *Table 1. The Vayus and Their Functions*: Table is based on Anderson, "The 5 Prana Vayus in Yoga," and oral teachings I received at the Yoga Studies Institute, Tucson, Arizona, in 2009–2010.

p. 65   *Table 2. The Chakras and Their Functions*: Table is based on A. Judith, *Wheels of Life*, and A. Mookerjee, *Kundalini: The Arousal of Inner Energy* (Inner Traditions, 1991).

p. 68   *As we practice, we generate prana*: Saraswati, *Surya Namaskara*, 3.

Week Four: Consciousness

p. 79   *"There is a vastness beyond"*: Sri Nisargadatta Maharaj, *I Am That*, 507.

p. 81   *The purpose of spiritual practice*: Easwaran, *The Bhagavad Gita*, 17.

p. 84   *"The wholehearted acceptance of pain"*: Sri Nisargadatta Maharaj, *I Am That*, 317.

p. 88   *"Anger is the response when attachment"*: Robina Courtin, "Is It Possible to Love without Attachment?," *Robina Courtin* (blog), March 4, 2019, https://robinacourtin.com/is-it-possible-to-love-without-attachment-2/.

p. 90   *"The soul always knows what to do"*: Caroline Myss, quoted in Enza DeLuca, *Blissful Mind, Blissful Body: Think Yourself Happier and Healthier* (Balboa Press, 2014), 13.

p. 96 *"will blossom into an all-pervading"*: Sri Nisargadatta Maharaj, *I Am That*, 508.

p. 98 *By redirecting our focus*: Gregg Braden, interview with André Duqum, "Becoming Superhuman: Unlock the Full Potential of Your Mind and Heart," episode of *Know Thyself* (podcast), YouTube video, 1:59:41, posted April 23, 2024, https://www.youtube.com/watch?v=3Zw-fA VO2Q4.

Week Five: Stories

p. 101 *"The story you tell yourself"*: Chris Hemsworth, quoted in *Limitless with Chris Hemsworth*, six-part television series directed by Darren Aronofsky (National Geographic, 2022).

p. 102 *The following teaching from Roopa Pai's commentary*: Roopa Pai, *The Vedas and Upanishads for Children* (Hachette India, 2019), 385.

p. 105 *The Bhagavad Gita teaches us*: Easwaran, *The End of Sorrow*, 102.

p. 107 *The Bhagavad Gita encourages us*: S. Radhakrishnan, *The Bhagavadgita* (HarperCollins, 2014), 80.

p. 114 *"Whatever follows 'I AM...'"*: Joel Osteen, interview with Oprah Winfrey, "The Two Powerful Words That Can Change Your Life," episode of *Oprah's Super Soul* (podcast), August 10, 2017.

Week Six: Mantra

p. 121 *"The mind binds us or frees us"*: Author's paraphrase from Easwaran, *The Upanishads*, 288.

p. 121 *we may experience impostor syndrome*: The term *impostor phenomenon* was introduced in 1978 in *Psychotherapy: Theory, Research, and Practice* in an article titled "The Impostor Phenomenon in High Achieving Women: Dynamics and Therapeutic Intervention" by Pauline R. Clance and Suzanne A. Imes. It has since been found to be experienced by people of all genders.

p. 122 *"Children are spending hours"*: Matt Platkin, quoted in "Dozens of States Sue Meta for Addictive Social Media Features Targeting Kids," *Democracy Now!*, October 25, 2023, https://www.democracynow.org/2023 /10/25/headlines/dozens_of_states_sue_meta_for_addictive_social _media_features_targeting_kids.

p. 128 *"Think of the power of the Universe"*: Charlie Chaplin, quoted in C. Sreechinth, *Chaplin for Thoughts: Greatest Quotes of King of Laugh* (UB Tech, 2016), 35.

p. 129 *positive statements can rewire*: Mayo Clinic Staff, "Positive Thinking: Stop
Negative Self-Talk to Reduce Stress," Mayo Clinic, https://www.mayo
clinic.org/healthy-lifestyle/stress-management/in-depth/positive-thinking
/art-20043950.

Week Seven: Choices

p. 136 *"On this path, effort never goes"*: Easwaran, *The Bhagavad Gita*, 93.
p. 137 *Those led by impatience*: Easwaran, *Essence of the Upanishads*, 42.
p. 139 *"Everything can be taken from a man"*: Viktor E. Frankl, *Man's Search for Meaning* (1959; repr., Beacon Press, 2006), 62.
p. 141 *"The Other is the one who taught me"*: Paulo Coelho, *By the River Piedra I Sat Down and Wept* (1996; repr., Harper, 1997), 50–51.

Week Eight: The Summit of Wisdom

p. 153 *"I am another you"*: Luís Valdez and Domingo Martinez Paredes, "In Lak'ech: You Are My Other Me," Guadalupe Carrasco Cardona (website), http://www.guadalupecardona.com/in-lak-ech.html.
p. 154 *"Deep in the heart of every creature"*: Easwaran, *The Upanishads*, 195.
p. 154 *I have realized the Self*: Easwaran, *The Upanishads*, 290.
p. 154 *The illumined ones serve love*: Easwaran, *The Upanishads*, 291–93.
p. 162 *ignorance of the interconnectedness*: S. Shahi and C. Rätsch, *Shamanism and Tantra in the Himalayas* (Inner Traditions, 2002).
p. 163 *"see the Self" in all beings*: Easwaran, *The Bhagavad Gita*, 128.
p. 163 *individuals in satisfying marriages*: T. F. Robles and J. K. Kiecolt-Glaser, "The Physiology of Marriage: Pathways to Health," *Physiology & Behavior* 79, no. 3 (August 2003): 409–16, https://doi.org/10.1016/S0031 -9384(03)00160-4.
p. 164 *evidence linking social relationships*: Sheldon Cohen, "Social Relationships and Health," *American Psychologist* 59, no. 8 (2004): 676–84, https://doi.org/10.1037/0003-066X.59.8.676.
p. 164 *"All paths lead to Me"*: Easwaran, *The Bhagavad Gita*, 117.
p. 165 *The word* Hindu *originates*: Pai, *The Vedas and Upanishads for Children*, 37–38.

Week Nine: Alchemy

p. 174 *"It is in giving that we receive"*: "St. Francis of Assisi: Make Me an Instrument of Your Peace," Archdiocese of Saint Pail & Minneapolis, accessed

November 1, 2024, https://www.archspm.org/faith-and-discipleship
/prayer/catholic-prayers/st-francis-of-assisi-make-me-an-instrument-of
-your-peace/.

p. 176   *"Purify yourself by a well-ordered"*: Sri Nisargadatta Maharaj, *I Am That*, 30.

Week Ten: Self-Healing

p. 210   *"what you bring forth will save the world"*: a theme in the Bhagavad Gita,
paraphrased in Stephen Cope, *The Great Work of Your Life: A Guide for
the Journey to Your True Calling* (Bantam, 2015), chaps. 3 and 18.

p. 211   *"You are what your deep"*: Easwaran, *The Upanishads*, 114.

Week Eleven: Meditation

p. 217   *A study from Harvard happiness experts*: Matthew A. Killingsworth and
Daniel T. Gilbert, "A Wandering Mind Is an Unhappy Mind," *Science*
330, no. 6006 (2010): 932, https://dtg.sites.fas.harvard.edu/KILLINGS
WORTH%20&%20GILBERT%20%282010%29.pdf; Jenifer Goodwin,
"Happiness Is a Focused Mind," HealthDay, December 16, 2010, Conscious Living Counseling and Education Center (website), https://www
.kamajensen.com/blog/uncategorized/happiness-is-focused-mind/#:~:-
text=If%20you%20want%20to%20be,in%20whatever%20they%20
were%20doing.

p. 218   *Meditation does it without*: Deepak Chopra, "7 Ways Meditation Can
Help You Reduce and Manage Stress," Presence (website), March 22,
2018, https://presence.app/blogs/meditation/7-ways-meditation-can
-help-you-reduce-and-manage-stress.

p. 220   *This theory is based on*: Deb Dana, *Polyvagal Theory in Therapy* (W. W.
Norton, 2018).

Week Twelve: Service and Celebration

p. 238   *"Consciousness is my home"*: Sri Nisargadatta Maharaj, *I Am That*, 507.

p. 240   *"Indian spirituality encompasses profound"*: Sri Sri Ravi Shankar, interview with Karishma Mehta, "Gurudev Sri Sri Ravi Shankar on Love,
Spiritual Knowledge, and Miracles," episode of *Realign* (podcast), You-
Tube video, 18:38, posted January 24, 2024, https://www.youtube.com
/watch?v=5lkrB23Wx-g&t=557s.

p. 242 *only those who have purified the mind*: Easwaran, *The Upanishads*, 144.

p. 246 *"You can't be what you can't see"*: Marian Wright Edelman, quoted in Esihle Makitshi, "You Can't Be What You Can't See," United Nations Institute for Training and Research, https://unitar.org/about/news-stories/stories/you-cant-be-what-you-cant-see.

p. 247 *Research indicates that recognizing*: Melanie A. McNally, "From Small Steps to Big Wins: The Importance of Celebrating," *Psychology Today*, June 12, 2024, https://www.psychologytoday.com/us/blog/empower-your-mind/202406/from-small-steps-to-big-wins-the-importance-of-celebrating.

p. 247 *Setting clear goals lays the foundation*: McNally, "From Small Steps."

ABOUT THE AUTHOR

Reema Datta is the founder of the Yogi's Way, a holistic method that integrates movement, breathing, and consciousness practices with a focus on emotional well-being. Since 2002, she has taught yoga trainings and retreats in over twenty countries across five continents. Reema is coauthor of the book *Sacred Sanskrit Words for Yoga, Chant, and Meditation* and has two mantra albums released by Nettwerk Music. Born into a family deeply rooted in yoga tradition, she was first taught by her parents and grandparents. She is a certified Ashtanga yoga and Tibetan heart yoga instructor and an Ayurvedic therapist. A graduate of Vassar College and the London School of Economics, Reema left her career working for the United Nations in 2001. Her students have included Sting, Edie Brickell, Paul Simon, Zainab Salbi, Sujatha Baliga, and thousands of other practitioners globally. Reema lives in Taos, New Mexico, with her daughter, Mila. For a schedule of her online and in-person trainings and events, see TheYogisWay.com.